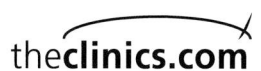

VETERINARY CLINICS OF NORTH AMERICA

Small Animal Practice

State of the Art Veterinary Oncology

GUEST EDITOR
Ruthanne Chun, DVM

November 2007 • Volume 37 • Number 6

SAUNDERS
An Imprint of Elsevier, Inc.
PHILADELPHIA LONDON TORONTO MONTREAL SYDNEY TOKYO

W.B. SAUNDERS COMPANY
A Division of Elsevier Inc.

Elsevier, Inc., 1600 John F. Kennedy Blvd., Suite 1800, Philadelphia, PA 19103-2899

http://www.vetsmall.theclinics.com

VETERINARY CLINICS OF NORTH AMERICA:	**Volume 37, Number 6**
SMALL ANIMAL PRACTICE	**ISSN 0195-5616**
November 2007	ISBN-13: 978-1-4160-5560-0
Editor: John Vassallo; j.vassallo@elsevier.com	ISBN-10: 1-4160-5560-6

Copyright © 2007 by Elsevier Inc. All rights reserved. No part of this publication may be reproduced or transmitted in any form or by any means, electronic or mechanical, including photocopy, recording, or any information retrieval system, without written permission from the Publisher.

Single photocopies of single articles may be made for personal use as allowed by national copyright laws. Permission of the publisher and payment of a fee is required for all other photocopying, including multiple or systematic copying, copying for advertising or promotional purposes, resale, and all forms of document delivery. Special rates are available for educational institutions that wish to make photocopies for non-profit educational classroom use. Permission may be sought directly from Elsevier's Global Rights Department in Oxford, UK: phone 215-239-3804 or +44 (0)1865 843830, fax +44 (0)1865 853333, e-mail healthpermissions@elsevier.com. Requests may also be completed online via the Elsevier homepage (http://www.elsevier.com/permissions). In the USA, users may clear permissions and make payments through the Copyright Clearance Center, Inc., 222 Rosewood Drive, Danvers, MA 01923, USA; phone: (978) 750-8400, fax: (978) 750-4744, and in the UK through the Copyright Licensing Agency Rapid Clearance Service (CLARCS), 90 Tottenham Court Road, London W1P 0LP, UK; phone: (+44) 171 436 5931; fax: (+44) 171 436 3986. Other countries may have a local reprographic rights agency for payments.

The ideas and opinions expressed in *Veterinary Clinics of North America: Small Animal Practice* do not necessarily reflect those of the Publisher. The Publisher does not assume any responsibility for any injury and/or damage to persons or property arising out of or related to any use of the material contained in this periodical. The reader is advised to check the appropriate medical literature and the product information currently provided by the manufacturer of each drug to be administered to verify the dosage, the method and duration of administration, or contraindications. It is the responsibility of the treating physician or other health care professional, relying on independent experience and knowledge of the patient, to determine drug dosages and the best treatment for the patient. Mention of any product in this issue should not be construed as endorsement by the contributors, editors, or the Publisher of the product or manufacturers' claims.

Veterinary Clinics of North America: Small Animal Practice (ISSN 0195-5616) is published bimonthly (For Post Office use only: volume 37 issue 6 of 6) by Elsevier Inc., 360 Park Avenue South, New York, NY 10010-1710. Months of issue are January, March, May, July, September, and November. Business and Editorial offices: 1600 John F. Kennedy Blvd., Suite 1800, Philadelphia, PA 19103-2899. Customer Service Office: 6277 Sea Harbor Drive, Orlando, FL 32887-4800. Periodicals postage paid at New York, NY and additional mailing offices. Subscription prices are $206.00 per year for US individuals, $327.00 per year for US institutions, $103.00 per year for US students and residents, $273.00 per year for Canadian individuals, $410.00 per year for Canadian institutions, $285.00 per year for international individuals, $410.00 per year for international institutions and $140.00 per year for Canadian and foreign students/residents. To receive student/resident rate, orders must be accompanied by name of affiliated institution, date of term, and the *signature* of program/residency coordinator on institution letterhead. Orders will be billed at individual rate until proof of status is received. Foreign air speed delivery is included in all *Clinics* subscription prices. All prices are subject to change without notice.
POSTMASTER: Send address changes to *Veterinary Clinics of North America: Small Animal Practice*, Elsevier Periodicals Customer Service, 6277 Sea Harbor Drive, Orlando, FL 32887-4800, USA; phone: 1-800-654-2452 [toll free number for US customers], or (+1)(407) 345-4000 [customers outside US]; fax: (+1)(407) 363-1354; email: usjcs@elsevier.com.

Veterinary Clinics of North America: Small Animal Practice is also published in Japanese by Inter Zoo Publishing Co., Ltd., Aoyama Crystal-Bldg 5F, 3-5-12 Kitaoyama, Minato-ku, Tokyo 107-0061, Japan.

Reprints: For copies of 100 or more, of articles in this publication, please contact the Commercial Reprints Department, Elsevier Inc., 360 Park Avenue South, New York, New York 10010-1710. Tel. (212) 633-3813 Fax: (212) 462-1935, email: reprints@elsevier.com.

Veterinary Clinics of North America: Small Animal Practice is covered in *Current Contents/Agriculture, Biology and Environmental Sciences, Science Citation Index, ASCA, Index Medicus, Excerpta Medica,* and *BIOSIS.*

Printed in the United States of America.

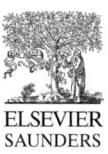

VETERINARY CLINICS
SMALL ANIMAL PRACTICE

State of the Art Veterinary Oncology

GUEST EDITOR

RUTHANNE CHUN, DVM, Diplomate, American College of Veterinary Internal Medicine (Oncology); Clinical Associate Professor, School of Veterinary Medicine, University of Wisconsin–Madison, Madison, Wisconsin

CONTRIBUTORS

PHILIP J. BERGMAN, DVM, MS, PhD, Diplomate, American College of Veterinary Internal Medicine (Oncology); Chief Medical Officer, Brightheart Veterinary Centers, Armonk; Adjunct Associate Faculty Member, Memorial Sloan-Kettering Cancer Center, New York, New York

BARBARA J. BILLER, DVM, PhD, Diplomate, American College of Veterinary Internal Medicine (Oncology); Assistant Professor of Oncology, Department of Clinical Sciences, College of Veterinary Medicine and Biomedical Sciences, Colorado State University, James L. Voss Veterinary Teaching Hospital, Fort Collins, Colorado

RUTHANNE CHUN, DVM, Diplomate, American College of Veterinary Internal Medicine (Oncology); Clinical Associate Professor, School of Veterinary Medicine, University of Wisconsin–Madison, Madison, Wisconsin

GREGORY B. DANIEL, DVM, MS, Professor and Head, Department of Small Animal Clinical Sciences, Virginia-Maryland Regional College of Veterinary Medicine, Virginia Polytechnic Institute and State University, Blacksburg, Virginia

TIMOTHY M. FAN, DVM, PhD, Diplomate, American College of Veterinary Internal Medicine; Assistant Professor of Medical Oncology, Department of Veterinary Clinical Medicine, University of Illinois at Urbana-Champaign, Urbana, Illinois

LISA J. FORREST, VMD, Diplomate, American College of Veterinary Radiology (Radiology, Radiation Oncology); Associate Professor of Radiology, Department of Surgical Sciences, University of Wisconsin–Madison, Madison, Wisconsin

LAURA D. GARRETT, DVM, Diplomate, American College of Veterinary Internal Medicine (Oncology); Clinical Assistant Professor, Small Animal Clinic, College of Veterinary Medicine, University of Illinois at Urbana-Champaign, Urbana, Illinois

CHAND KHANNA, DVM, PhD, Diplomate, American College of Veterinary Internal Medicine (Oncology); Director, Tumor Metastasis and Biology Section, Comparative Oncology Program, National Cancer Institute, National Institutes of Health, Bethesda, Maryland

CONTRIBUTORS continued

JESSICA A. LAWRENCE, DVM, Diplomate, American College of Veterinary Radiology (Radiation Oncology); Medical Oncology Resident, Department of Medical Sciences, University of Wisconsin–Madison, Madison, Wisconsin

AMY K. LeBLANC, DVM, Assistant Professor of Oncology, Department of Small Animal Clinical Sciences, College of Veterinary Medicine, University of Tennessee, Knoxville, Tennessee

CHERYL A. LONDON, DVM, PhD, Diplomate, American College of Veterinary Internal Medicine (Oncology); Shackelford Professor of Veterinary Medicine; and Associate Professor, Department of Veterinary Biosciences, College of Veterinary Medicine, The Ohio State University, Columbus, Ohio

ANTHONY J. MUTSAERS, DVM, Diplomate, American College of Veterinary Internal Medicine (Oncology); Terry Fox Foundation Post-Doctoral Fellow, National Cancer Institute of Canada; Division of Molecular and Cell Biology, Sunnybrook Health Sciences Centre, Department of Medical Biophysics, University of Toronto, Toronto, Ontario, Canada

MELISSA C. PAOLONI, DVM, Diplomate, American College of Veterinary Internal Medicine (Oncology); Comparative Oncology Program, National Cancer Institute, National Institutes of Health, Bethesda, Maryland

DAVID M. VAIL, DVM, Diplomate, American College of Veterinary Internal Medicine (Oncology); Professor of Oncology; and Director, Center for Clinical Trials and Research, School of Veterinary Medicine, University of Wisconsin–Madison, Madison, Wisconsin

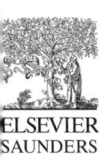

VETERINARY CLINICS
SMALL ANIMAL PRACTICE

State of the Art Veterinary Oncology

CONTENTS VOLUME 37 • NUMBER 6 • NOVEMBER 2007

Preface xi
Ruthanne Chun

Communicating with Oncology Clients 1013
Ruthanne Chun and Laura D. Garrett

Empathic, honest, and consistent communications that establish realistic goals and focus on quality of life (during and after therapy) for pets with cancer provide the basis of an excellent client-veterinarian relationship. From this foundation, a client can team up with his or her veterinarian to make the best possible decisions for the pet and for himself or herself regarding care for the companion animal.

Comparative Oncology Today 1023
Melissa C. Paoloni and Chand Khanna

The value of comparative oncology has been increasingly recognized in the field of cancer research, including the identification of cancer-associated genes; the study of environmental risk factors, tumor biology, and progression; and, perhaps most importantly, the evaluation of novel cancer therapeutics. The fruits of this effort are expected to be the creation of better and more specific drugs to benefit veterinary and human patients who have cancer. The state of the comparative oncology field is outlined in this article, with an emphasis on cancer in dogs.

Cancer Clinical Trials: Development and Implementation 1033
David M. Vail

Although much of the current standard of care in veterinary oncology is based on retrospective studies or transference from the human literature, a new era of clinical trial awareness brought on by new consortia and cooperative investigative groups is beginning to change this limitation. The use of controlled, randomized, blind multicenter trials testing new cytotoxics and cytostatic agents is now becoming the norm rather than the exception. Ultimately, advanced clinical trial design applied to companion animal populations should advance veterinary-based practice and inform future human clinical trials that may follow.

Advanced Imaging for Veterinary Cancer Patients 1059
Amy K. LeBlanc and Gregory B. Daniel

This article presents an update on the recent advances made in veterinary advanced imaging specifically with regard to cross-sectional modalities (CT and MRI) and nuclear medicine (positron emission tomography [PET] and PET/CT). A brief summary of technical improvements and a review of recent literature are included to provide an overview of the progress made in this important element of the practicing veterinary oncologist's repertoire. An in-depth summary of PET is also included to introduce the technical aspects and potential clinical and research applications of this novel imaging modality in veterinary medicine.

Chemotherapy: New Uses for Old Drugs 1079
Anthony J. Mutsaers

Using chemotherapy drugs as antiangiogenic agents is a new use for drugs that have been around for a long time. The favorable toxicity profile and reduced cost make low-dose continuous "metronomic" chemotherapy trials appealing, but there is still much to be learned. Challenges ahead include determination of the optimal tumor types, drugs, doses, schedules, and response monitoring (end points). The measurement of angiogenic growth factors and inhibitors and of circulating endothelial progenitor cells or their precursors represents promising strategies in these areas.

The Role of Bisphosphonates in the Management of Patients That Have Cancer 1091
Timothy M. Fan

Bisphosphonates are pharmacologic agents widely used in people for managing pathologic bone resorptive conditions. Based on their physicochemical properties, bisphosphonates concentrate within areas of active bone remodeling and induce osteoclast apoptosis. Appropriate use of bisphosphonates for treating companion animals requires a thorough understanding of how bisphosphonates exert their biologic effects. This review article highlights general properties of bisphosphonates, including their pharmacology, mechanisms of action, adverse side effects, anticancer mechanisms, surrogate markers for assessing response, and potential clinical utility for treating dogs and cats diagnosed with malignant skeletal tumors.

Anticancer Vaccines 1111
Philip J. Bergman

With the tools of molecular biology and a greater understanding of mechanisms to harness the immune system, effective tumor immunotherapy is becoming a reality. This new class of therapeutics offers a more targeted, and therefore precise, approach to the treatment of cancer. The recent conditional licensure of a xenogeneic DNA vaccine for advanced canine malignant melanoma strongly suggests that immunotherapy can play an

CONTENTS continued

extremely important role alongside the classic cancer treatment triad components of surgery, radiation therapy, and chemotherapy.

The Role of Small Molecule Inhibitors for Veterinary Patients 1121
Cheryl A. London

Advances in molecular biology over the past several years have permitted a much more detailed understanding of cellular dysfunction at the biochemical level in cancer cells. This has resulted in the identification of novel targets for therapeutic intervention, including proteins that regulate signal transduction, gene expression, and protein turnover. In many instances, small molecules are used to disrupt the function of these targets, often through competitive inhibition of ATP binding or the prevention of necessary protein-protein interactions. Future challenges lie in identifying appropriate targets for intervention and combining small molecule inhibitors with standard treatment modalities, such as radiation therapy and chemotherapy.

Cancer Immunotherapy for the Veterinary Patient 1137
Barbara J. Biller

The ability of the immune system to protect against tumor development and to attack malignant cells once they arise has been recognized for more than 50 years. Since this time, our understanding of the complex relation between the immune system and the development of cancer has increased dramatically, largely because of improvements in the tools used to study tumor immunology at the molecular level. These advances are leading to the development of increasingly sophisticated and effective immunotherapeutics for human and veterinary oncology patients; indeed, some forms of immunotherapy already have a place alongside more conventional treatment modalities, such as surgery, radiation therapy, and chemotherapy.

Intensity-Modulated Radiation Therapy and Helical Tomotherapy: Its Origin, Benefits, and Potential Applications in Veterinary Medicine 1151
Jessica A. Lawrence and Lisa J. Forrest

Intensity-modulated radiation therapy (IMRT), especially image-guided IMRT as represented by helical tomotherapy, is a novel approach to therapy and is rapidly evolving. Both of these forms of therapy aim to allow targeted radiation delivery to the tumor volume while minimizing dose to the surrounding normal tissues. Adaptive radiation therapy and conformal avoidance are possible with intensity-modulated therapy and helical tomotherapy, which offer opportunities for improved local tumor control, decreased normal tissue toxicity, and improved survival and quality of life. Human and veterinary patients are likely to benefit from the continued development of this radiation delivery technique, and data over the next several years should be crucial in determining its true benefit.

Index **1167**

VETERINARY CLINICS
SMALL ANIMAL PRACTICE

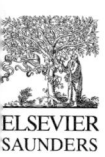

FORTHCOMING ISSUES

January 2008
    Oxidative Stress, Mitochondrial Dysfunction, and Novel Therapies
    Lester Mandelker, DVM
    Guest Editor

March 2008
    Ophthalmic Immunology and Immune-Mediated Disease
    David L. Williams, MA, VetMB, PhD
    Guest Editor

May 2008
    Advances in Fluid, Electrolyte, and Acid-Base Disorders
    Helio Autran de Morais, DVM, PhD and Stephen P. DiBartola, DVM
    Guest Editors

RECENT ISSUES

September 2007
    Respiratory Physiology, Diagnostics, and Disease
    Lynelle R. Johnson, DVM, MS, PhD
    Guest Editor

July 2007
    The Thyroid
    Cynthia R. Ward, VMD, PhD
    Guest Editor

May 2007
    Evidence-Based Veterinary Medicine
    Peggy L. Schmidt, DVM, MS
    Guest Editor

THE CLINICS ARE NOW AVAILABLE ONLINE!

Access your subscription at:
http://www.theclinics.com

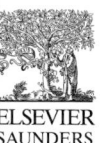

Preface

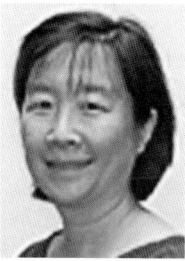

Ruthanne Chun, DVM
Guest Editor

When invited to be guest editor of this issue, I was excited to be able to showcase some of the opportunities that are available at referral institutions and in practice. Now, more than ever, veterinary oncologists have the double satisfaction of helping individuals and helping science. Although some view oncology as a "dead end" specialty, those who practice it know that they are making a difference to animals and their owners on a daily basis. Although the recent January 2007 issue of *Veterinary Clinics of North America: Small Animal Practice* was devoted entirely to veterinary communication skills, Laura Garrett and I thought that there are enough communication issues specific to oncology to warrant an article on this topic. As has been so clearly demonstrated in human medicine and is now being documented in veterinary practice, good client communication skills and a trusting client-veterinarian relationship result in better adherence to treatment recommendations, greater client satisfaction, and less professional burnout for the doctor.

Most of this issue is devoted to advances in veterinary oncology. The knowledge base that supports our understanding of cancer is growing, and veterinary medicine is poised to play a key role in the development of better diagnostics and therapeutics. Melissa Paoloni and Chand Khanna explain how veterinary oncology is now giving valuable information back to human oncology in their article entitled "Comparative Oncology Today." In addition to helping human patients who have cancer, clinical trials that benefit veterinary patients are becoming more and more common. David Vail describes the important mechanics behind the planning and execution of a clinical trial in "Cancer Clinical Trials: Development and Implementation." Amy LeBlanc and Greg Daniel discuss how diagnostic imaging options are rapidly expanding as radiologists are using functional imaging studies not only to stage disease but to monitor response to treatment and adjust therapy as necessary.

Other important areas of state-of-the-art new treatment options are described by Tony Mutsaers, Cheryl London, Tim Fan, Barbara Biller, and Phil Bergman. From new ways to use existing chemotherapy drugs, to using small molecule inhibitors designed to aim at specific targets on or surrounding cancer cells, to immunotherapy and anticancer vaccines, this issue describes the changes that are encompassing medical oncology.

Finally, an exciting cutting-edge radiation therapy modality is described by Jessica Lawrence and Lisa Forrest. Although use of this technology is just gaining popularity in human radiation oncology, we are excited to announce that tomotherapy will be available at the University of Wisconsin–Madison School of Veterinary Medicine starting in 2009.

Thus, although some things in veterinary oncology may never change (like the use of the cyclophosphamide, hydroxydaunorubicin [doxorubicin], Oncovin [vincristine], prednisone protocol for lymphoma), there are many advances happening in veterinary oncology. I hope that this issue makes those changes clear and puts them within the grasp of the practitioner.

Ruthanne Chun, DVM
School of Veterinary Medicine
University of Wisconsin-Madison
2015 Linden Drive
Madison, WI 53706, USA

E-mail address: chunr@svm.vetmed.wisc.edu

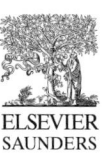

Communicating with Oncology Clients

Ruthanne Chun, DVM[a],*, Laura D. Garrett, DVM[b]

[a]School of Veterinary Medicine, University of Wisconsin–Madison, 2015 Linden Drive, Madison, WI 53706, USA
[b]Small Animal Clinic, College of Veterinary Medicine, University of Illinois at Urbana-Champaign, 1008 W Hazelwood Dr., Urbana, IL 61802, USA

Good communication skills are recognized as a cornerstone of successful veterinary practice [1]. A concise compilation of effective communication techniques for veterinarians has been published recently [2]. Although strong communication skills are essential for all veterinarians, oncology, in particular, requires that the clinician be able to engage and empathize with his or her clients. Oncology patients undergoing chemotherapy or radiation therapy require frequent visits to the veterinarian, and timing of therapy is critical. Thus, clients must be thoroughly educated regarding the logistics, side effects, and costs of their pets'quo; therapy, and they must adhere to the prescribed treatment protocol to maximize therapeutic efficacy. Thus, the recently espoused "4E" model of engagement, empathy, education, and enlistment is particularly pertinent to the veterinary oncologist [3,4]. Clients can be empowered through appropriate engagement and enlistment into the management of their pet's disease, and this can result in better adherence to prescribed treatment regimens and follow-up visits [5]. Further, multiple studies in the field of human oncology have identified effective communication skills as a source of satisfaction for the patient and the clinician [6–10].

REVIEW OF BASIC COMMUNICATION SKILLS

Because of the relatively sparse formal communication training in most veterinary curriculums, the authors start with a review of basic communication skills. A well-crafted interview is essential for obtaining a thorough and accurate history. One of the most important aspects of effective communication is attending not only to what is being said but how it is being said. Communication has verbal and nonverbal components. Although it is stated that as much as 80% of what is actually communicated depends on nonverbal factors (eg, facial expression, posture, eye contact, intonation) [11], initial factual information must be gathered through the history and physical examination. Specific interviewing techniques, such as open- and close-ended questions,

*Corresponding author. E-mail address: chunr@svm.vetmed.wisc.edu (R. Chun).

paraphrasing, reflective listening and summarizing (Table 1), can be used to gather an accurate and complete history. The use of these skills can also affect the client's perception of the veterinarian. The veterinarian must also be aware of his or her own nonverbal cues and those of the client for the best communication and patient care to occur.

The initial minutes of an appointment heavily influence the veterinary-client relationship. As initially described by Strong's Social Influence Theory, the combination of expertness, trustworthiness, and attractiveness can be conceptualized as an equilateral triangle (Fig. 1) [12]. The veterinarian must convey expertness (eg, knowledge of veterinary medicine), trustworthiness (eg, open

Table 1
Examples of interviewing techniques

Questioning skill	Goal	Example
Open-ended question	Request elaboration on a specific point. Allows client to provide frame of reference	How has Fritzie been doing since her last treatment?
Close-ended question	A way to obtain specific data or point clarification, limit discussion topic, or focus client	Did Fritzie have any vomiting or diarrhea?
Paraphrasing	Ensures accurate clinician understanding of the client's statements	It sounds like she starting vomiting 3 days after her treatment and she has vomited at least four times a day since then.
	A powerful way to emphasize the importance of a specific point	
Summarizing	Essentially a paraphrase of the entire history or a recapitulation of the plan	Because of the prolonged vomiting, beyond what I would have expected as a result of chemotherapy, I would like to check Fritzie out with some blood work and abdominal ultrasound to try to determine the cause of her stomach upset.
Reflective listening	Directly acknowledges what the client just said	You're saying that Fritzie's chemotherapy side effects have been unacceptable.
Empathic statement	Acknowledges client emotion	It can be hard to see a companion become ill after a treatment.

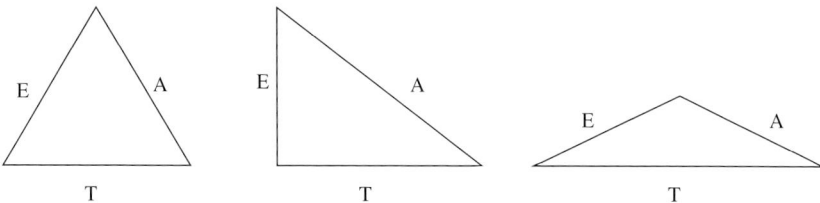

Fig. 1. Balance, or lack thereof, in client perception of expertness (E), trustworthiness (T), and attractiveness (A).

body posture, eye contact), and attractiveness (eg, expression of empathy, ability to interact well with the pet). Clients have different needs; some may want only high levels of expertness without regard for attractiveness, whereas others desire a strong demonstration of attractiveness before they feel comfortable in leaving their companion for diagnostic testing and treatment. Further, veterinarians may need to vary their own communication style depending on the client [4]. A collaborative approach, with the veterinarian educating the client about the disease and then working together with the client to come up with the best plan for the patient, is advocated. This approach results in a client who is invested as a part of a team providing health care for the pet and leads to increased trust in the veterinarian and increased compliance on the part of the client. Other roles the veterinarian can take on are as "guardian" or "teacher." In the guardian role, the veterinarian presents the owner not only with the diagnosis but with what is to be done next diagnostically and therapeutically, without the owner's input. A potential major disadvantage of the guardian role is that an adverse outcome is more likely to be blamed on the veterinarian, who made all the decisions. In the teacher role, the veterinarian presents an owner with all the scientific information available regarding the disease, further tests, and treatment options but does not help the client in applying that information to his or her pet and situation. A potential major disadvantage of the teacher role is that the client may feel frustrated by his or her inability to decipher the best option and may seek opinions at other veterinary clinics.

BREAKING THE NEWS/PRESENTING THE DIAGNOSIS

Clients need time to adjust to the idea that their pet may have a terminal illness. Small "sound bites" work best when advising an owner that there may be a malignant process involved. Mentioning the possibility of cancer as one of the differentials before a definitive diagnosis has its pros and cons. Although it is important to avoid inducing unnecessary worry and fear by the suggestion of cancer, it can be helpful to prepare an owner for that diagnosis when the likelihood of such a finding is high. Being up-front about a neoplastic differential can help an owner to adjust to the idea and deal with the diagnosis in a more coherent and proactive manner once it is confirmed.

Once the diagnosis is made, it is important to keep the information provided about the disease on a basic level initially. Even with prior warning that the diagnosis could be cancer, some clients may be shocked by the diagnosis and may only be able to take in small bits of what is said, such as: "Unfortunately, the results have come back as lymphoma. This is one of the most common cancers we see in dogs. The good news is that it is treatable, but, unfortunately, it is not curable. Would you like to discuss further testing and treatment options now, or would you prefer that we talk later?"

Keep in mind that clients and clinicians may have baggage associated with the terms *cancer* and *chemotherapy*. The initial response to the diagnosis may alter as the pet owner accepts the results and hears more about the condition. An initial refusal to consider any more testing or treatment often changes with further education about how well most dogs and cats do with their cancer therapy. Giving the client time to adjust and asking for permission to provide more information can help with the owner's transition from grief over the diagnosis to taking an active role in making treatment choices for the pet.

RESPONDING TO CLIENT EMOTION

Even to the brave of heart, strong client emotions can be daunting [13]. A common concern is whether the client's emotion, once acknowledged, is going to escalate. In actuality, it is more common for the opposite to occur. The use of empathy, defined in this capacity as the recognition and comprehension of another's emotional situation, is a powerful tool. The ability to "stand in someone else's shoes" is especially important with oncology clients. Empathy does not mean that you feel what the client feels; it simply means that you can try to imagine how the situation would be from the client's point of view. Verbally acknowledging a client's distress helps the client to know that his or her feelings are seen, and thus helps to validate those feelings and to create a stronger client-veterinarian bond. A statement as simple as "I can see this is difficult for you; it can be very hard to hear that someone so close to you has cancer" can be grounding for a client and may allow him or her to refocus on the medical discussion.

OFFERING OPTIONS

One of the key aspects to helping clients through the diagnosis and treatment of their companion animal is to be open and honest in the information provided and to do so in the language of the client. Explaining things in "layperson's" terms is always important in communication with a pet owner, but it becomes even more critical in the highly charged discussions surrounding a diagnosis of cancer. Clients can easily become overwhelmed with the news of the diagnosis and may be too distraught or embarrassed to stop the veterinarian and ask for explanations about words they do not understand. After years in training and medical practice, it is easy to forget that commonly used terminology, such as renal, radiograph, and injection, may not be understood by the average pet owner. A conscious effort to use such words as kidney, x-ray, and shot instead can help an owner to stay with the conversation, and thus lead to better care for the patient in the end.

Oftentimes, a diagnosis of cancer can be made after only limited testing, such as an aspirate of an oral mass revealing melanoma. Staging, or evaluating for the systemic extent of a cancer, is critical in making further treatment decisions and in more accurately predicting the prognosis for the patient. Much can be discussed with an owner given the initial diagnosis, however, before any other testing. In a dog with oral melanoma, for example, the biologic behavior (eg, locally aggressive, highly metastatic), the treatment options, and the rough prognosis based on size of the mass are known and can be presented to the owner. Recommendations for further indicated tests (eg, lymph node aspirates, thoracic radiographs) and explanations of their associated costs and what they may reveal (eg, how likely it is to find metastatic disease with a certain tumor type) can all be covered in the first meeting after the diagnosis is made. Clients can then make educated decisions regarding the pursuit of further tests or therapies. Some owners are able to make a decision not to treat based on this first discussion alone, and they appreciate the veterinarian not running a barrage of tests that would not make a difference in their decision-making process in the end. Other owners may have set finances available and may have to decline noncritical tests to be able to afford their pet's therapy (eg, thoracic and abdominal radiographs for staging lymphoma may not be performed so that the client can afford more chemotherapy treatments).

In discussing treatment options for a pet with cancer, it is important to present a range of options yet even more important not to overwhelm an owner with too many choices. In situations in which there is a therapy that has clearly been shown to provide the best results, it is appropriate to present that therapy first as the most effective option. Costs (short term and long term), logistics (eg, how many hospital visits are needed), and potential side effects need to be presented in detail verbally and in writing. If the "gold standard" therapy is declined, other treatment options can be presented, also with their associated costs, logistics, and side effects.

It is critical to say that choosing not to treat is always a reasonable decision. Owners may have many reasons for this choice, and the veterinarian's support is important. Some owners may decide not to treat based on misconceptions surrounding cancer and its therapy, however. Thus, educating the owner on how well companion animals tolerate most medical, surgical, and radiation therapies used against tumors is also critical. For example, explaining that more than 75% of dogs treated with chemotherapy have no side effects and that most of the remaining 25% that may have side effects can be handled at home may change an owner's decision about treatment. Another reason why an owner may choose not to treat is a poor prognosis. The critical issue here is to understand that the value of the additional time that treatment may provide for a client and his or her companion animal can be determined only by the client. Thus, "poor" in regard to prognosis is a relative term. Some owners think that an additional year of life is not a good enough prognosis, whereas others are grateful to have their pet an extra month or 2 months. It is important for the veterinarian to provide the objective data available in regard to treatments and prognoses, without imposing his or her own feelings about the value of that gain in survival time.

PROVIDING SUPPORT

As veterinarians, we are often called on to help support our clients through difficult decisions and, ultimately, the loss of their companion. Many animals are treasured members of the family. Additionally, pets can have special significance to their owners, having helped them through a difficult time or being a final link to a deceased loved one. The authors have experienced multiple situations in which the animal's original owner died (often of cancer) and the animal itself is now being lost to cancer. The value of a trusting physician-patient relationship has been reported; the patient's ability to cope is enhanced, and there is a reduced probability of malpractice litigation and professional burnout [9]. Although less documentation exists for veterinary medicine, the same principles can apply. Although veterinarians are not mental health professionals, showing empathy and being a "good listener" are important skills [14] and are especially important with oncology clients. An empathic veterinary team, in addition to support from personal relationships, can help most clients to get through the difficulty of losing a pet. Some clients need more help, however. It is important to know mental health professionals in the area who understand the grief that can surround pet loss and are willing to counsel clients experiencing difficulty. Letting clients know that you are concerned about them and providing names or business cards of local counselors can be expressed in a variety of ways. Examples of ways to discuss referral to a mental health professional include the following:

- I can see how hard this situation is for you. I'm wondering if it would be helpful for you to speak with someone who can help you more than I can. I have worked with a counselor who has been helpful with some of my clients. Would you like her business card?
- You have had such a difficult time, not just with Fritzie but with so many other things. Have you considered talking to a counselor or someone who can provide you with support?
- I'm worried about you. Do you have someone that you can talk to so you can get through this more easily?

One common and often frustrating aspect of communicating with oncology clients is the frequent occurrence of "second-guessing" the veterinarian's recommendations. One common example is the client who contacts multiple veterinary clinics or uses the Internet excessively to gather opinions and options. This "bargaining" for a better outcome is a well-recognized stage of grief. Although especially difficult in some situations, it is important to remain open but consistent with these clients. Some comments that might be useful in such a situation are included in Table 2. A different example of when consistency is

Table 2
Examples of how to respond to a client's second-guessing of your recommendations

Client comment	Veterinary response
Dr. Jones told me that they always use drug X with great success in these cases.	I am recommending the best known care for Muffy. I understand that you want to leave no stone unturned, and if you want to try less well-known treatment options, we can do that.
Don't you think that she could be one of the dogs who is cured?	I would love it if Muffy was cured of this disease. Keep in mind that her odds of cure are slim, but I don't want to tell you there is no hope.

needed is when an aggressive cancer responds well to therapy in the short term and the client "forgets" the long-term outlook and repeatedly asks whether the pet is cured. The authors have experienced clients who resorted to asking technicians and office staff if the pet was cured in spite of (or perhaps because of) the veterinarian's consistent reply that it was extremely unlikely. Although it would often be easier just to agree with the owner, staying realistic and consistent about the prognosis ultimately leads to a more satisfying result for all, because an owner with unrealistic expectations may be disappointed and dissatisfied in the end.

Another example in which consistency of the long-term prognosis is important is when there are complications of the disease or its treatment, or if other conditions arise. Weighing expected survival times associated with the tumor being treated can become important when another life-threatening and expensive or intensive new problem arises. Some clients would opt to support their cat being treated for relapsed lymphoma through the uncommon complication of sepsis secondary to chemotherapy-induced myelosuppression. Others would opt for surgery to correct gastric dilatation and volvulus in a dog with osteosarcoma and small pulmonary metastasis. Although the cancer could lead to their death in the near future in both of these patients, many clients choose to treat the more immediate threat, and thus prolong their pet's life as long as possible. Although some might view this decision as a waste of money in a situation with no good long-term outlook, it is the authors'quo; opinion that quality of life is the bottom line. In other words, it may be reasonable to pursue aggressive treatments if the patient has a good chance of returning to a normal quality of life for a time, the value of which is purely the client's decision.

END-OF-LIFE DECISIONS

Veterinary medicine is not unique in performing euthanasia. In states in which the death penalty is legal, convicted criminals may be put to death. The association of euthanasia as the ultimate punishment or, at minimum, with "giving up" can be extremely difficult for people to get past. The concept of euthanasia as a "final gift" and a release from suffering associated with a terminal disease should be openly discussed. In a study reporting results of a survey of 177 clients regarding the death of their pet, even though 84% responded that euthanasia was a good option to end their pet's life humanely, up to 50% of clients felt guilty or questioned whether they made the right decision for their pet, 16% said they felt like a murderer, and 30% experienced severe grief [15].

Because of the negative stigma associated with cancer, it is easier for clients to understand that their pet may have an incurable disease. Throughout this article, the authors have emphasized that clients must be educated in regard to the diagnosis, treatment options, and expected quality of life and prognosis. In keeping with this theme, it is equally important to discuss the option of euthanasia with clients. The "right time" varies from client to client, with some choosing euthanasia before quality of life worsens at all and others waiting until quality of life is unacceptable. Ideally, clients should consider their "bottom-line" quality-of-life issues and changes days to months before the final decision may need to be made. Because of the human-animal bond, pets may always come to greet them at the door, wag their tails, or ask for a caress. Telephone interviews with clients owning cats with cancer identified poor quality of life, perceived suffering, and lack of cure as the top reasons for selecting euthanasia [16]. Thus, an emphasis on quality-of-life issues (eg, the pet's ability to urinate/defecate on its own, eat anything, do activities it previously enjoyed) is most helpful in guiding clients. Most clients are able to make the decision to euthanize at the time that is right for them and their pet.

Clients must also decide what to do with their pet's body. Typical options include disposal through clinic services, burial, and group or private cremation. Some clients may request donation of their pet's body for teaching purposes (some veterinary schools have donation programs for their anatomy laboratories) or necropsy. Common motivations expressed include the desire to have something positive (eg, learning) come from their pet's death and interest in knowing the extent of disease at the time of death.

EUTHANASIA

The authors prefer witness euthanasias to those performed in a treatment room with no client present. Not all clients want to be with their pet at the time of death, however. Experiencing euthanasia may be one of the most profound moments in a client's life. During a witness euthanasia procedure, the client may share private information or display unusual behavior attributable to grief. Again, the veterinary team should provide as supportive and empathic an environment as possible. As mentioned previously in this article, acknowledgment of and, especially in the case of grief, validation of strong client emotion is an aspect that clients find particularly important [15].

Ideally, witness euthanasia should be performed in a quiet room during a less busy time of day for the clinician. Clients should be gently informed of the euthanasia process. Many clients are unaware of how rapidly animals die after injection of euthanasia solution. Body changes, such as loss of bladder or bowel control, the eyes remaining open, and reflexive sighs or twitching, can be distressing or even shocking to pet owners. Warning of these potential occurrences can greatly alleviate the distress or fear that a client may feel should such things happen. An intravenous catheter placed in a rear leg (usually placed in the treatment area away from the owner) provides direct venous access for injection and allows the client to be at the pet's head during the procedure. Placing the catheter ahead of time guarantees smooth intravenous access and also allows the owner to know that his or her pet does not even feel a needle at the time of injection. After the injection is complete and the heartbeat has stopped, some owners want to have time alone, whereas others do not. Visiting with the owner about his or her pet immediately after the euthanasia procedure can be helpful for the owner and the veterinary team in dealing with the loss. Discussing favorite memories of the pet can be a way of celebrating the life of the loved one. Also, a follow-up telephone call or sympathy card is a good way to let the owner know that he or she and the pet are remembered and that others are thinking of them. Well-performed euthanasia is an invaluable medical procedure, and good communication surrounding the event is key to a smooth outcome and a grateful client [17].

Empathic, honest, and consistent communications that establish realistic goals and focus on quality of life (during and after therapy) for pets with cancer provide the basis of an excellent client-veterinarian relationship. From this foundation, a client can team up with his or her veterinarian to make the best possible decisions for the pet and for himself or herself regarding care for the companion animal.

References

[1] Frankel RM. Pets, vets, and frets: what relationship-centered care research has to offer veterinary medicine. J Vet Med Educ 2006;33(1):20–7.

[2] Cornell KK, Brandt JC, Bonvicini KA. Effective communication in veterinary practice. Philadelphia: W.B. Saunders; 2006. Vet Clin North Am Small Anim Pract; vol. 37.

[3] Keller VF, Carroll JG. A new model for physician-patient communication. Patient Educ Couns 1994;23:131–40.

[4] Cornell KK, Kopcha M. Client-veterinarian communication: skills for client centered dialogue and shared decision making. Vet Clin North Am Small Anim Pract 2007;37(1):37–47.

[5] Abood SK. Increasing adherence in practice: making your clients partners in care. Vet Clin North Am Small Anim Pract 2007;37(1):151–64.

[6] Armstrong J, Holland J. Surviving the stresses of clinical oncology by improving communication. Oncology 2004;18(3):363–8.

[7] Baile WF, Aaron J. Patient-physician communication in oncology: past, present, and future. Curr Opin Oncol 2005;17(4):331–5.

[8] Lienard A, Merckaert I, Libert Y, et al. Factors that influence cancer patients' anxiety following a medical consultation: impact of a communication skills training programme for physicians. Ann Oncol 2006;17(9):1450–8.

[9] Bredart A, Bouleuc C, Dolbeault S. Doctor-patient communication and satisfaction with care in oncology. Curr Opin Oncol 2005;17(4):351–4.

[10] Delvaux N, Merckaert I, Marchal S, et al. Physicians' communication with a cancer patient and a relative: a randomized study assessing the efficacy of consolidation workshops. Cancer 2005;103(11):2397–411.

[11] Carson CA. Nonverbal communication in veterinary practice. Vet Clin North Am Small Anim Pract 2007;37(1):49–63.

[12] Strong SR. Counseling: an interpersonal influence process. J Couns Psychol 1968;15(3): 215–24.
[13] Tinga CE, Adams CL, Bonnett BN, et al. Survey of veterinary technical and professional skills in students and recent graduates of a veterinary college. J Am Vet Med Assoc 2001;219(7): 924–31.
[14] Martin EA. Managing client communication for effective practice: what skills should veterinary graduates have acquired for success? J Vet Med Educ 2006;33(1):45–9.
[15] Adams CL, Bonnett BN, Meek AH. Predictors of owner response to companion animal death in 177 clients from 14 practices in Ontario. J Am Vet Med Assoc 2000;217(9):1303–9.
[16] Slater MR, Barton CL, Rogers KS, et al. Factors affecting treatment decisions and satisfaction of owners of cats with cancer. J Am Vet Med Assoc 1996;208(8):1248–52.
[17] Martin F, Ruby KL, Deking TM, et al. Factors associated with client, staff, and student satisfaction regarding small animal euthanasia procedures at a veterinary teaching hospital. J Am Vet Med Assoc 2004;224(11):1774–9.

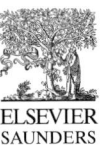

Comparative Oncology Today

Melissa C. Paoloni, DVM, Chand Khanna, DVM, PhD*

Comparative Oncology Program, National Cancer Institute, National Institutes of Health, 37 Convent Drive, Room 2144, Bethesda, MD 20892, USA

Comparative oncology is an approach that has recently gained significant prominence in the lay and scientific press [1–3]. Comparative oncology refers to the discipline that integrates the naturally occurring cancers seen in our veterinary patients into more general studies of cancer biology and therapy. This includes the study of cancer pathogenesis (ie, the study of cancer-associated genes and proteins) and the study of new treatment options for the management of cancer [4]. By nature, this approach provides novel opportunities for current and future veterinary and human patients who have cancer. Although several veterinary species, including the cat, horse, and ferret, develop cancers that are of comparative interest, most of the scientific and clinical effort has thus far focused on the dog [5]. This is attributable to the strong anatomic and physiologic similarities between dogs and human beings, their long use as a toxicologic model in drug development, and, most importantly, the sheer number of dogs that are diagnosed and managed with cancer annually [1,4,6–10]. The state of the comparative oncology field is outlined in this article, with an emphasis on cancer in dogs.

PROBLEM OF CANCER IN DOGS

The problem of cancer in dogs is a serious challenge that we face as veterinarians. It is estimated that one in four dogs greater than 2 years of age dies of cancer, and certain popular breeds are overrepresented in terms of cancer incidence and mortality [1,4,6]. The prevalence of cancer in dogs has increased in recent years. This may be the result of an actual increase in cancer incidence, an increase in the population of dogs at risk for the development of cancer, or the awareness and interest in the pet-owning community to pursue diagnostic and treatment options. Advances in the care of animals have allowed dogs to live longer because of better nutrition, vaccination for common infectious diseases, leash laws that limit automobile deaths, and the availability of more sophisticated diagnostics and treatments for many ailments previously considered to be life-threatening. The improved general health of pets has resulted in an

*Corresponding author. E-mail address: khannac@mail.nih.gov (C. Khanna).

0195-5616/07/$ – see front matter
doi:10.1016/j.cvsm.2007.08.003

Published by Elsevier Inc.
vetsmall.theclinics.com

increase in age-related diseases, including cancer. Aware of the treatment options available for two-legged family members, pet owners now demand advanced care options for four-legged family members diagnosed with cancer. This includes all traditional treatment modalities, such as surgery, radiation therapy, immunotherapy, and chemotherapy, and novel investigational drugs available through participation in clinical trials [4,11–28].

COMPARATIVE ADVANTAGE

Cancer in dogs shares with cancer in human beings many features, including histologic appearance, tumor genetics, molecular targets, biologic behavior, and response to conventional therapies (Fig. 1) [1–4,17,29–46]. Significantly, cancer develops naturally in dogs within the environment they share with their human owners. Tumor initiation and progression are influenced by similar factors, including age, nutrition, gender, reproductive status, and environmental exposures [9,47]. The spectrum of cancers seen in dogs is as diverse as that seen in human patients. Some histologies of comparative interest include osteosarcoma, melanoma, non-Hodgkin's lymphoma, leukemia, prostate

Comparative Oncology

INTEGRATES NATURALLY OCCURRING CANCER MODELS IN THE STUDY OF CANCER BIOLOGY AND THERAPY

Cancer in Companion Animals
- 70 Million Companion Dogs in the US
- 1-6 million pet dogs diagnosed with cancer each year
- Pet owners seek advanced care for their pets

Attributes

- Spontaneously Occurring
- Strong Genetic Similarities to Humans
- Immune Competent
- Relevant Tumor Histologies and Genetics
- Relevant Response Chemotherapy
- No "Standards of Care"
- Compressed Progression Times
- Tumor Heterogeneity
- Metastasis Biology
- Recurrence/Resistance

Fig. 1. Advantages of comparative oncology. Cancer is a prevalent disease in dogs. The pet-owning public is highly motivated to seek advanced care for pets and is interested in traditional and experimental therapies. Comparative oncology aims to use the dog as a sophisticated model for the study of cancer biology and therapy. Attributes of this opportunity are numerous. Cancer in dogs naturally shares many of the genetic aberrations, oncogene overexpression, and tumor suppressor loss seen in the human disease. This provides a platform for the evaluation of target biology. Importantly, pet dogs with cancer capture the complexity of cancer by representing tumor heterogeneity within individual tumors and between patients with the same diagnosis in a way impossible in traditional research models, thus allowing for the study of metastasis biology, disease recurrence, and resistance patterns in true clinical patients, corresponding to the key elements of the problem of cancer in human beings.

carcinoma, mammary carcinoma, lung carcinoma, head and neck carcinomas, soft tissue sarcomas, and bladder carcinoma.

More important than histologic appearance, the basic biology of cancer in dogs is similar to that of cancer in human beings. Most, if not all, of the cancer-associated genetic alterations that influence cancer progression in human beings have been identified in canine cancer [3,6,34,36,38,40,42–44,48,49]. Many of the chemotherapy protocols used in veterinary medicine were originally co-opted from protocols used to treat human patients and have a similar activity spectrum [4]. For example, the same chemotherapeutics that are active in canine lymphoma are those active in human lymphoma (ie, vincristine, cyclophosphamide, doxorubicin, mitoxantrone, cytarabine arabinoside, methotrexate) [4]. The opposite is also true; the drugs not as helpful in canine lymphoma are also not as helpful in human lymphoma (ie, gemcitabine, cisplatin, carboplatin) [4]. Similar parallels have been seen in investigative and targeted therapeutics. The biologic complexity of cancers in pet animals mirrors that of the human disease, based largely on the intratumoral (cell-to-cell) heterogeneity seen in these cancers. Natural consequences of this heterogeneity are the deadly features of all cancers, which include acquired resistance, recurrence, and metastasis [1,2,4,9,31,50,51]. In these ways, companion animal cancers capture the "essence" of the problem of cancer in ways not seen in other animal model systems.

A WINDOW OF OPPORTUNITY

The opportunity to expand the scope of questions asked and answered through a comparative oncology approach has been the result of the completion of the recent canine genome sequence and resultant technologies generated using this genetic information. The efforts of the Canine Genome Project have resulted in the 2005 public release of a high-quality sequence covering 99% of the canine genome (2.5 billion base pairs) [31,33]. Interrogation of the genome sequence suggests that all the approximately 19,000 genes identified in the dog match to similar or orthologous genes in the human genome [31,33]. Thus, the genome of the dog and the genome of the human being are similar enough to suggest that information learnt about one species can be transferred to and applicable to the other. The information provided by the canine genome sequence has become increasingly usable to veterinarians and research scientists through reductions in the costs for development of scientific tools [32,52,53]. For example, oligonucleotide microarrays have been available for the study of gene expression in human and murine tissues for several years. This technology allows the assessment of thousands, and soon millions, of gene segments within a single tissue in a matter of hours. The availability of a well-described canine genome has now led to the development of commercially available canine expression microarrays. Therefore, veterinary cancers can be increasingly described in the same "language" as their human counterparts. This infrastructure provides the ability to conduct detailed and biologically intensive studies in canine cancer not previously possible, which can evaluate target genes/proteins and pathways important in cancer biology, study their changes after exposure to new cancer therapies (described as pharmacodynamics), and connect the changes in these cancer targets to successful therapy.

The exploratory tools now available for the study of canine cancer have also been useful in studying the causes of human and canine caners. Unfortunately, dogs of all breeds, including the ever-popular mixed breed, develop cancer. It has been known for many years, however, that there are some breeds with a higher incidence of cancer. This has been an emphasis of research funding by the Morris Animal Foundation (MAF) and the American Kennel Club–Canine Health Foundation (AKC-CHF) [6,50]. Some overrepresented breeds include the boxer for mast cell tumors, rottweilers and greyhounds for osteosarcoma, golden retrievers for lymphoma, Scottish terriers for transitional cell carcinoma of the bladder, flat-coated retrievers and Bernese mountain dogs for histiocytic sarcomas, and chow chows for melanoma [4,31,48,54]. Interestingly, decreased cancer incidence has also been reported in some breeds as well. Studying breeds with increased cancer incidence is potentially informative because the breed lines of most dogs are known with historically well-documented pedigrees. Predisposed breeds provide the platform to identify genes known to be linked to cancer development (ie, oncogenes) and those whose loss triggers cancer development or progression (ie, tumor suppressor genes). Several genetic alterations and molecular signaling pathways known to be important in human cancers have been defined and shown to be relevant in canine cancers [3,6,34,36,38,40,42–44,49]. The genetic similarities between dogs within a breed may allow more rapid progress in the identification of new cancer-associated genes than the study of human or mouse cancers alone.

OPPORTUNITIES PROVIDED TO PETS BY THE COMPARATIVE APPROACH

Clinical trials in veterinary oncology are increasing in number and scope. Attributes of the comparative approach are a considerable reason for this increase because they provide a unique opportunity to integrate studies that include dogs with cancer into the development path of new cancer drugs [3,12,13,15–18,21,23,26,37,55]. These new drugs may be used in dogs with cancer before or during their study in human patients. The ability to gather serial biopsies from tumors and repeated fluid collections (eg, serum, plasma, whole blood, urine) from the same patient during exposure to an investigational agent can answer complex questions about how best to use drugs that cannot be answered from tumor measurements alone (Fig. 2). This serial sampling allows for the identification of tumor and surrogate markers of drug activity or target modulation, pharmacodynamic end points, which can be uniquely correlated to response in ways that are often not feasible in traditional preclinical rodent studies or in human cancer trials.

Interest from the human cancer drug development industry is based on a need for more reliable ways to evaluate new cancer drugs and the strong similarities established between veterinary and human cancers [56,57]. Because

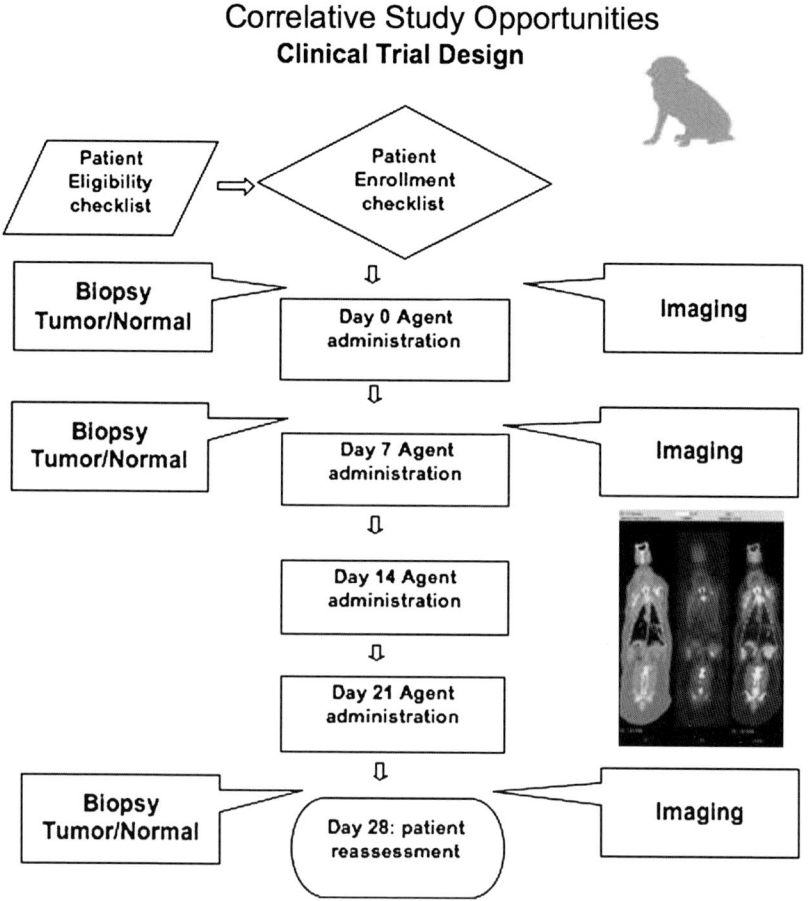

Fig. 2. Comparative oncology focused clinical trial design. Comparative oncology clinical trial designs focus on answering specific questions important for optimal drug development. The opportunity for serial biopsy of tumor, normal tissues, and other biofluids before, during, and after exposure to new agents is readily incorporated into study designs. Biologic evaluation of these tissues/samples can now include gene expression analysis, single nucleotide polymorphism (SNP) and comparative genomic hybridization (CGH) array genomics, and all protein-based analyses common in human studies. These evaluations can occur in parallel with advanced imaging studies, including CT, MRI, positron emission tomography (PET), and PET/CT. Thus, these studies allow for the unique correlation of drug exposure to tissue and fluid biomarkers and dynamic imaging end points. The anticipation is that studies in pet dogs can improve the efficiency of toxicologic assessment and also have the potential to evaluate biology and activity in a naturally occurring tumor model.

there are no treatment standards for the management of cancer in dogs, there is an added opportunity to provide pet owners and their dogs with access to novel therapeutics earlier in the course of disease and before treatment with conventional chemotherapy as compared with human patients participating in early-phase human cancer trials. Beyond the access to new and potentially effective treatments for cancer, most clinical trials involve targeted cancer treatments that are less likely to be associated with side effects than conventional treatment. Furthermore, trials often provide significant financial support to study participants. As such, studies are particularly appealing to populations of clients who would otherwise forego traditional cancer treatments. The naturally shorter life span of our patients also permits the more rapid completion of clinical trials of novel agents that can assess outcome within a 6- to 18-month window, again impossible in human cancer trials. The benefits of such clinical trials in dogs include earlier assessment of drug activity and toxicity critical to the design of more informed future veterinary and human clinical trials.

Several cooperative groups exist to study cancer in dogs. These organizations are made up of veterinary oncologists, surgeons, geneticists, basic scientists, and general practitioners who wish to understand the causes of cancer in dogs, seek improved treatments, and use the dog as a comparative model. The American College of Veterinary Internal Medicine [58] is the body responsible for training board-certified veterinary specialists in medical oncology. The American College of Veterinary Radiology [59] trains individuals to become board-certified in radiation oncology. The Veterinary Cancer Society (VCS) [60], founded in 1977, is an organization focused on education and the sharing of scientific knowledge within the veterinary oncology community. The VCS, along with the Veterinary Co-Operative Oncology group (VCOG), has encouraged multicenter collaborative studies that have largely been retrospective in nature. In 2006, the Comparative Oncology and Genomics Consortium (CCOGC) [61], a new not-for-profit entity, was established. The CCOGC consists of a broad representation of parties focused on the genetics and biology of cancer naturally occurring in dogs. A primary effort of the CCOGC has been the development of a canine cancer biospecimen repository that can provide materials for large-scale studies of canine cancer biology.

The Comparative Oncology Program (COP) [62] of the National Cancer Institute was developed in 2003 and has established a multicenter collaborative network of academic comparative oncology programs known as the Comparative Oncology Trials Consortium (COTC). The COTC is made up of 14 veterinary teaching hospitals, and the goal of this effort is to conduct well-organized and focused clinical trials that provide biologically rich answers to the cancer therapeutic development pathway. These trials emphasize pharmacokinetic and pharmacodynamic end points, correlating drug exposure to modulation of tumoral markers and defining their relation to activity. The first two COTC trials were conducted at seven different institutions. COTC001 involved systemic delivery of a targeted phage carrying the gene for tumor necrosis factor-α (TNFα), a known potent cytotoxic and antiangiogenic agent that has been difficult to administer safely in the past. Data from a preliminary study showed that this novel delivery method could effectively target tumor vasculature and spare normal organs while identifying a safely tolerable dose. These data were used to design a second study in which the agent was given once weekly and its effect on response was measured. COTC001 was illustrative of the benefits of the comparative approach, because the drug's target was unique to tumor vasculature. Pet dogs with cancer were a necessary model to demonstrate the targeting specificity of this agent within a naturally heterogeneous tumor environment. This model provided the ability to evaluate fully the potential toxicities and efficacy of this drug, which would not have been equally achieved in more traditional research models. Information from this trial is currently directing the development path of this drug for human patients who have cancer. COTC003 involves the evaluation of rapamycin in dogs with osteosarcoma, a drug that inhibits an important oncogenic pathway called mTOR, which is upregulated in many tumor types. Again, the approach in the first phase of study is to define a dose that may be safely administered to dogs and that is capable of effectively inhibiting the activated mTOR pathway within the tumor and perhaps correlating to a secondary blood marker of this activity. A follow-up study in dogs plans to measure rapamycin's benefit as a treatment for metastatic osteosarcoma. COTC003 provides an example of the benefits of serial tissue sampling, allowing for evaluation of a target pathway before and after exposure to a new drug. This type of information is vital to designing more successful second-phase treatment trials in canine and human patients who have cancer and is impossible to accomplish uniformly in trials in people. Also, both phases of this study are scheduled to be completed in less than 1.5 years, which is much faster than the comparable human trials with analogues of this drug. This provides an opportunity for early and simultaneous reporting of canine data and subsequent integration of pertinent findings within the ongoing human clinical trials. If effective, this drug holds promise for future development in both species. As illustrated by both of these trials, information provided by COTC studies aims to improve the drug development pathway by answering critical questions regarding how best to use novel agents for the treatment of cancer in dogs and people.

All the multicenter efforts described emphasize collaborative science to integrate comparative oncology further into mainstream studies of cancer biology. Most clinical trials are conducted through academic veterinary teaching hospitals or referral centers but, increasingly, include direct involvement from general practitioners. Engaging general practitioners in the conduct of comparative oncology trials is essential to their success. This encourages more robust patient accrual, compliant client participation, and more accurate outcome and toxicity reporting.

SUMMARY

The value of comparative oncology has been increasingly recognized in the field of cancer research, including the identification of cancer-associated genes; the study of environmental risk factors, tumor biology, and progression; and, perhaps most importantly, the evaluation of novel cancer therapeutics. Like all innovations, it is important to define when the comparative oncology approach should and should not be used. This should continuously be defined on an agent or target basis and evaluated as this approach is used in the future.

The fruits of this effort are expected to be the creation of better and more specific drugs to benefit veterinary and human patients who have cancer.

References

[1] Khanna C, Lindblad-Toh K, Vail D, et al. The dog as a cancer model. Nat Biotechnol 2006;24(9):1065–6.
[2] Vail DM, MacEwen EG. Spontaneously occurring tumors of companion animals as models for human cancer. Cancer Invest 2000;18(8):781–92.
[3] Hansen K, Khanna C. Spontaneous and genetically engineered animal models; use in preclinical cancer drug development. Eur J Cancer 2004;40(6):858–80.
[4] Withrow SJ, Vail DM. Withrow & MacEwen's small animal clinical oncology. 4th edition. St. Louis (MO): Saunders Elsevier; 2007.
[5] Antinoff N, Hahn K. Ferret oncology: diseases, diagnostics, and therapeutics. Vet Clin North Am Exot Anim Pract 2004;7(3):579–625, vi.
[6] Olson PN. Using the canine genome to cure cancer and other diseases. Theriogenology 2007;68(3):378–81.
[7] Naylor RJ, Rudd JA. Mechanisms of chemotherapy/radiotherapy-induced emesis in animal models. Oncology 1996;53(Suppl 1):8–17.
[8] Bukowski JA, Wartenberg D, Goldschmidt M. Environmental causes for sinonasal cancers in pet dogs, and their usefulness as sentinels of indoor cancer risk. J Toxicol Environ Health A 1998;54(7):579–91.
[9] Hahn KA, Bravo L, Adams WH, et al. Naturally occurring tumors in dogs as comparative models for cancer therapy research. In Vivo 1994;8(1):133–43.
[10] Mutsaers AJ, Widmer WR, Knapp DW. Canine transitional cell carcinoma. J Vet Intern Med 2003;17(2):136–44.
[11] Rusk A, McKeegan E, Haviv F, et al. Preclinical evaluation of antiangiogenic thrombospondin-1 peptide mimetics, ABT-526 and ABT-510, in companion dogs with naturally occurring cancers. Clin Cancer Res 2006;12(24):7444–55.
[12] Rusk A, Cozzi E, Stebbins M, et al. Cooperative activity of cytotoxic chemotherapy with antiangiogenic thrombospondin-I peptides, ABT-526 in pet dogs with relapsed lymphoma. Clin Cancer Res 2006;12(24):7456–64.
[13] Thamm DH, Kurzman ID, King I, et al. Systemic administration of an attenuated, tumor-targeting Salmonella typhimurium to dogs with spontaneous neoplasia: phase I evaluation. Clin Cancer Res 2005;11(13):4827–34.
[14] Buchholz J, Kaser-Hotz B, Khan T, et al. Optimizing photodynamic therapy: in vivo pharmacokinetics of liposomal meta-(tetrahydroxyphenyl)chlorin in feline squamous cell carcinoma. Clin Cancer Res 2005;11(20):7538–44.
[15] Vail DM, Amantea MA, Colbern GT, et al. Pegylated liposomal doxorubicin: proof of principle using preclinical animal models and pharmacokinetic studies. Semin Oncol 2004;31(6 Suppl 13):16–35.
[16] London CA, Hannah AL, Zadovoskaya R, et al. Phase I dose-escalating study of SU11654, a small molecule receptor tyrosine kinase inhibitor, in dogs with spontaneous malignancies. Clin Cancer Res 2003;9(7):2755–68.
[17] Khanna C, Vail DM. Targeting the lung: preclinical and comparative evaluation of anticancer aerosols in dogs with naturally occurring cancers. Curr Cancer Drug Targets 2003;3(4):265–73.
[18] Khanna C, Prehn J, Hayden D, et al. A randomized controlled trial of octreotide pamoate long-acting release and carboplatin versus carboplatin alone in dogs with naturally occurring osteosarcoma: evaluation of insulin-like growth factor suppression and chemotherapy. Clin Cancer Res 2002;8(7):2406–12.
[19] MacEwen EG, Kurzman ID, Vail DM, et al. Adjuvant therapy for melanoma in dogs: results of randomized clinical trials using surgery, liposome-encapsulated muramyl tripeptide, and

granulocyte macrophage colony-stimulating factor. Clin Cancer Res 1999;5(12): 4249–58.
[20] Hershey AE, Kurzman ID, Forrest LJ, et al. Inhalation chemotherapy for macroscopic primary or metastatic lung tumors: proof of principle using dogs with spontaneously occurring tumors as a model. Clin Cancer Res 1999;5(9):2653–9.
[21] Khanna C, Waldrep JC, Anderson PM, et al. Nebulized interleukin 2 liposomes: aerosol characteristics and biodistribution. J Pharm Pharmacol 1997;49(10):960–71.
[22] Vail DM, MacEwen EG, Kurzman ID, et al. Liposome-encapsulated muramyl tripeptide phosphatidylethanolamine adjuvant immunotherapy for splenic hemangiosarcoma in the dog: a randomized multi-institutional clinical trial. Clin Cancer Res 1995;1(10): 1165–70.
[23] Kurzman ID, MacEwen EG, Rosenthal RC, et al. Adjuvant therapy for osteosarcoma in dogs: results of randomized clinical trials using combined liposome-encapsulated muramyl tripeptide and cisplatin. Clin Cancer Res 1995;1(12):1595–601.
[24] Kurzman ID, Cheng H, MacEwen EG. Effect of liposome-muramyl tripeptide combined with recombinant canine granulocyte colony-stimulating factor on canine monocyte activity. Cancer Biother 1994;9(2):113–21.
[25] Withrow SJ, Thrall DE, Straw RC, et al. Intra-arterial cisplatin with or without radiation in limb-sparing for canine osteosarcoma. Cancer 1993;71(8):2484–90.
[26] LaRue SM, Withrow SJ, Powers BE, et al. Limb-sparing treatment for osteosarcoma in dogs. J Am Vet Med Assoc 1989;195(12):1734–44.
[27] Elmslie RE, Dow SW. Genetic immunotherapy for cancer. Semin Vet Med Surg (Small Anim) 1997;12(3):193–205.
[28] Dow SW, Potter TA. Expression of bacterial superantigen genes in mice induces localized mononuclear cell inflammatory responses. J Clin Invest 1997;99(11):2616–24.
[29] Sutter NB, Bustamante CD, Chase K, et al. A single IGF1 allele is a major determinant of small size in dogs. Science 2007;316(5821):112–5.
[30] Patrick DJ, Fitzgerald SD, Sesterhenn IA, et al. Classification of canine urinary bladder urothelial tumours based on the World Health Organization/International Society of Urological Pathology consensus classification. J Comp Pathol 2006;135(4):190–9.
[31] Ostrander EA, Giger U, Lindblad-Toh K. The dog and its genome. Cold Spring Harbor (NY): Cold Spring Harbor Laboratory Press; 2006.
[32] Thomas R, Scott A, Langford CF, et al. Construction of a 2-Mb resolution BAC microarray for CGH analysis of canine tumors. Genome Res 2005;15(12):1831–7.
[33] Lindblad-Toh K, Wade CM, Mikkelsen TS, et al. Genome sequence, comparative analysis and haplotype structure of the domestic dog. Nature 2005;438(7069):803–19.
[34] Lee CH, Kim WH, Lim JH, et al. Mutation and overexpression of p53 as a prognostic factor in canine mammary tumors. J Vet Sci 2004;5(1):63–9.
[35] Jones CL, Grahn RA, Chien MB, et al. Detection of c-kit mutations in canine mast cell tumors using fluorescent polyacrylamide gel electrophoresis. J Vet Diagn Invest 2004;16(2): 95–100.
[36] Thomas R, Smith KC, Ostrander EA, et al. Chromosome aberrations in canine multicentric lymphomas detected with comparative genomic hybridisation and a panel of single locus probes. Br J Cancer 2003;89(8):1530–7.
[37] Pryer NK, Lee LB, Zadovaskaya R, et al. Proof of target for SU11654: inhibition of KIT phosphorylation in canine mast cell tumors. Clin Cancer Res 2003;9(15):5729–34.
[38] Lingaas F, Comstock KE, Kirkness EF, et al. A mutation in the canine BHD gene is associated with hereditary multifocal renal cystadenocarcinoma and nodular dermatofibrosis in the German Shepherd dog. Hum Mol Genet 2003;12(23):3043–53.
[39] Ozaki K, Yamagami T, Nomura K, et al. Mast cell tumors of the gastrointestinal tract in 39 dogs. Vet Pathol 2002;39(5):557–64.
[40] Lee CH, Kweon OK. Mutations of p53 tumor suppressor gene in spontaneous canine mammary tumors. J Vet Sci 2002;3(4):321–5.

[41] Wakui S, Muto T, Yokoo K, et al. Prognostic status of p53 gene mutation in canine mammary carcinoma. Anticancer Res 2001;21(1B):611–6.
[42] Setoguchi A, Sakai T, Okuda M, et al. Aberrations of the p53 tumor suppressor gene in various tumors in dogs. Am J Vet Res 2001;62(3):433–9.
[43] Reguera MJ, Rabanal RM, Puigdemont A, et al. Canine mast cell tumors express stem cell factor receptor. Am J Dermatopathol 2000;22(1):49–54.
[44] London CA, Galli SJ, Yuuki T, et al. Spontaneous canine mast cell tumors express tandem duplications in the proto-oncogene c-kit. Exp Hematol 1999;27(4):689–97.
[45] Van Leeuwen IS, Hellmen E, Cornelisse CJ, et al. P53 mutations in mammary tumor cell lines and corresponding tumor tissues in the dog. Anticancer Res 1996;16(6B):3737–44.
[46] London CA, Kisseberth WC, Galli SJ, et al. Expression of stem cell factor receptor (c-kit) by the malignant mast cells from spontaneous canine mast cell tumours. J Comp Pathol 1996;115(4):399–414.
[47] Hayes HM Jr, Fraumeni JF Jr. Epidemiological features of canine renal neoplasms. Cancer Res 1977;37(8 Pt 1):2553–6.
[48] Modiano JF, Breen M, Burnett RC, et al. Distinct B-cell and T-cell lymphoproliferative disease prevalence among dog breeds indicates heritable risk. Cancer Res 2005;65(13): 5654–61.
[49] Kiupel M, Webster JD, Kaneene JB, et al. The use of KIT and tryptase expression patterns as prognostic tools for canine cutaneous mast cell tumors. Vet Pathol 2004;41(4):371–7.
[50] Olson PN. Fighting cancer in dogs. J Am Vet Med Assoc 2007;230(9):1280–97.
[51] Porrello A, Cardelli P, Spugnini EP. Oncology of companion animals as a model for humans. An overview of tumor histotypes. J Exp Clin Cancer Res 2006;25(1):97–105.
[52] Lana S, Plaza S, Hampe K, et al. Diagnosis of mediastinal masses in dogs by flow cytometry. J Vet Intern Med 2006;20(5):1161–5.
[53] Lana SE, Jackson TL, Burnett RC, et al. Utility of polymerase chain reaction for analysis of antigen receptor rearrangement in staging and predicting prognosis in dogs with lymphoma. J Vet Intern Med 2006;20(2):329–34.
[54] Proschowsky HF, Rugbjerg H, Ersboll AK. Mortality of purebred and mixed-breed dogs in Denmark. Prev Vet Med 2003;58(1–2):63–74.
[55] MacEwen EG, Kurzman ID, Helfand S, et al. Current studies of liposome muramyl tripeptide (CGP 19835A lipid) therapy for metastasis in spontaneous tumors: a progress review. J Drug Target 1994;2(5):391–6.
[56] Kamb A, Wee S, Lengauer C. Why is cancer drug discovery so difficult? Nat Rev Drug Discov 2007;6(2):115–20.
[57] Kola I, Landis J. Can the pharmaceutical industry reduce attrition rates? Nat Rev Drug Discov 2004;3(8):711–5.
[58] Available at: www.acvim.org.
[59] Available at: www.acvr.org.
[60] Available at: www.vetcancersociety.org.
[61] Available at: ccr.cancer.gov/resources/cop/scientists/resource_genomics.asp.
[62] Available at: ccr.cancer.gov/resources/cop.

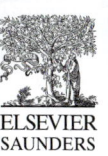

Cancer Clinical Trials: Development and Implementation

David M. Vail, DVM

Center for Clinical Trials and Research, School of Veterinary Medicine, University of Wisconsin-Madison, 2015 Linden Drive, Madison, WI 53706, USA

Although much of the current standard of care in veterinary oncology is based on retrospective studies or transference from the human literature, a new era of clinical trial awareness brought on by new consortia and cooperative investigative groups is beginning to change this limitation. The use of controlled, randomized, blind multicenter trials testing new cytotoxics and cytostatic agents is now becoming the norm rather than the exception. Ultimately, advanced clinical trial design applied to companion animal populations should advance veterinary-based practice and inform future human clinical trials that may follow.

Clinical trials represent a special kind of cohort study in which interventions are specifically introduced by the investigators in ways to improve the possibility of observing effects that are free of bias. The basic structure of clinical trials is represented in Fig. 1, and the specific type of clinical trial is defined by modifications of the basic component parts, namely, patient selection, treatment allocation, intervention, and outcome measurement. The ultimate goal of any clinical trial is to improve on the currently available standard of care. Although this review only deals with prospective clinical trials, unfortunately, a significant proportion of the standard of care in veterinary oncology is still based on retrospective data. It is important to state that retrospective studies should only be used to create questions that can be answered in prospective trials and rarely should the standard of care be changed based on the results of a retrospective analysis. Thankfully, more and more pharmaceutic agents are being developed specifically for companion animals licensure, and several pharmaceutical companies are seeking companion animal licensure of currently available off-label drugs; therefore, our reliance on retrospective data and the anthropomorphic translation of data from human trials is becoming less and less common.

In veterinary medicine, an additional goal of clinical trials is to contribute to and inform human clinical trials; that is, to use companion animal species with naturally occurring cancers for proof-of-principle or proof-of-concept trials that

E-mail address: vaild@svm.vetmed.wisc.edu

0195-5616/07/$ – see front matter © 2007 Elsevier Inc. All rights reserved.
doi:10.1016/j.cvsm.2007.06.007 vetsmall.theclinics.com

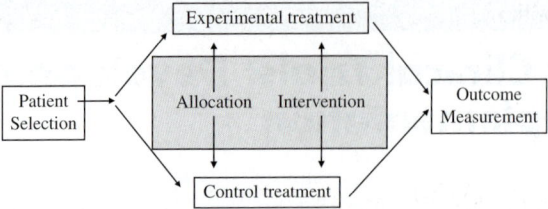

Fig. 1. Basic structure of clinical trials. The specific type of clinical trial is defined by modifications of the basic component parts, namely, patient selection, treatment allocation, intervention, and outcome measurement.

advance novel therapeutics or novel drug delivery techniques. Several recent editorials in the scientific press have attested to the model potential of companion animals, and the newly formed Comparative Oncology Trials Consortium at the National Cancer Institute has just completed the first of several clinical trials to help inform future human trials [1–4]. Ultimately, it is hoped that advancements made using companion animal species can advance the practice of veterinary oncology.

Careful planning and implementation are critical to the success of any trial, and this review seeks to take the reader through the various stages of anticancer drug development, discussing the traditional trial phases (I–IV) and exposing the reader to some alternative trial design modifications that are currently being evaluated or implemented. Several examples from the veterinary literature are used to illustrate trial design. One point of clarification is that several of the examples from the literature using companion animal species are published as "preclinical" studies because of the fact that physician-based oncology views veterinary data as such; however, as first-in-species veterinary trials, they are indeed "clinical" studies in the eyes of the veterinary profession. Additionally, an appendix is included with definitions to help the reader (Appendix I).

Several reviews in the human cancer literature have addressed the difficulties in advancing new drugs or therapies in the oncology realm [5–9]. It is estimated that only 5% to 10% of drugs entering phase I clinical trials ultimately get to market, with a cost of between 0.8 and 1.7 billion dollars per drug through development [10,11]. Oncology has one of the poorest records for drug development, with success rates more than three times lower than that for cardiovascular drugs [5,6]. There is therefore a tremendous need to improve the efficiency and speed of drug development, because too many patients and resources are used in one trial at the expense of other treatments, ultimately slowing medical progress [8]. The problem is further complicated by insisting on investigating newer molecular-targeted cytostatic agents using trial designs developed for traditional cytotoxic drugs. Indeed, it is estimated that more than 40% of drugs currently under development are targeting novel targets [9]. This represents a switch from a primary focus on toxicity to one of identifying a dose that optimally inhibits a specific target [5]; that is, the biologically optimal dose (BOD) may not relate to the maximally tolerated dose (MTD), a dose that is the more traditional starting point for efficacy trials. This also means that availability of validated assays of target modulation is becoming more and more important in the successful implementation of clinical trials for static targeted agents.

For the reader seeking more thorough reviews on design and statistical methods, recent reviews are listed throughout this article. Importantly, this article concerns itself with clinical trial design and implementation and not with statistical analysis of generated data. It cannot be stressed enough that all trial designs be thoroughly reviewed by a knowledgeable biostatistician to ensure that statistical design and power are appropriate before implementation.

TRADITIONAL DRUG DEVELOPMENT FLOW

Traditionally, first-in-species trials start with a phase I dose-finding trial, followed by a phase II efficacy/activity trial, and conclude with a phase III "comparative" trial that pits the novel agent against or with the current standard of care. The goals and salient points on each phase are summarized in Table 1.

Phase I Trials (Dose-Finding)

Phase I trial design and statistical considerations have been reviewed [5,12,13]. The primary goal of phase I trials is to determine the MTD to be used in future phase II studies by evaluating safety, tolerance, and dose-limiting toxicity (DLT) in treatment cohorts of increasing dose. Activity/efficacy is not a primary

Table 1
Goals of phase I through III clinical trials

Characteristic	Phase I (dose finding)	Phase II (activity/efficacy)	Phase III (comparative)
Primary goals	• Determine MTD • Define DLT • Elucidate parameters of toxicity	• Determine activity/efficacy in defined populations • Inform the decision to move to a phase III trial	• Compare a new drug or combination with therapy currently regarded as standard of care
Secondary goals	• PK/PD issues • Scheduling issues • Target modulation effects • Preliminary efficacy data	• Estimate therapeutic index • Expand toxicity data • Evaluate additional dosing groups • Expand target modulation data • Quality-of-life measures	• Quality-of-life comparisons • Comparative costs

Abbreviations: DLT, dose-limiting toxicity; PK/PD, pharmacokinetic/pharmacodynamic.

goal of phase I trials. In fact, response rates in phase I trials are seldom more than 10% [12]. This is particularly important with respect to informed consent, because even though clients are informed that they may be receiving a drug with nonexistent activity or at a suboptimal dose in early dosing groups, a full 50% of human subjects entering phase I trials believe they are going to experience a response [12]. Secondary goals of phase I trials may include scheduling issues, response rate, pharmacokinetic (PK) information (absorption, distribution, metabolism, and elimination [ADME]), and effects on molecular targets or pathways.

Who enters phase I trials?
In human oncology, the type of individual who enters a phase I trial is one who is refractory to standard of care. As such, subjects are generally heavily pretreated and have advanced disease and poor performance status (ie, significantly ill because of significant tumor burden or prior treatment effects). In veterinary medicine, the phase I patient may have failed standard of care, no effective standard of care exists, or the standard of care is beyond the financial wherewithal of the client. For example, several currently ongoing veterinary trials conducted by the clinical trials group at the University of Wisconsin offer treatment at reduced cost or also have financial assets in place that can be used by clients for standard of care should the novel test therapy prove ineffective in their companion animal. This is truly a win-win situation in many respects for the clients.

Setting the starting dose
Generally, some preclinical data exist (in other than the target species), and those data are used to inform a starting dose for phase I [5,7,12]. If other species (eg, rodent) toxicity data exist, one third of the "no observable adverse event level" (NOAEL) or one tenth of the severe toxicity dose in the most sensitive species is used to start with. If normal laboratory dog (usually Beagle dogs) data are available, the author has found over the years that it is prudent to start at 50% of the MTD in Beagles because they seem to be less sensitive to toxicity than tumor-bearing patient dogs. If the starting dose is too low, the length of the trials is longer, there is poor use of resources, and the number of patients exposed to suboptimal doses is increased. Some patient advocate groups are allowing patients to pick a starting dose based on varying degrees of risk; that is, some patients are willing to risk more toxicity for a higher likelihood of activity.

Dose escalation strategies
As with starting dose, escalation strategies greatly affect the number of patients treated at a potential ineffective dose, the length of the trial, and the risk of toxicity. The traditional method of escalation (Table 2) uses a "3 + 3" cohort design, wherein dose escalations are made with three dogs per dose level and the MTD is set based on the number of patients experiencing a DLT [5,12,13]. A DLT is defined as grade III or greater toxicity in any category (except hematologic) according to predefined adverse event categories, such as those in

Table 2
Standard phase I dose escalation scheme

No. patients with DLT at a given dose level	Escalation decision rule
0 of 3	Enter 3 patients at the next dose level
>2	Dose escalation will be stopped. This dose level will be declared the maximally administered dose (highest dose administered). Three (3) additional patients will be entered at the next lowest dose level if only 3 patients were treated previously at that dose.
1 of 3	Enter at least 3 more patients at this dose level. • If 0 of these 3 patients experience DLT, proceed to the next dose level. • If 1 or more of this group suffer DLT, then dose escalation is stopped, and this dose is declared the maximally administered dose. Three (3) additional patients will be entered at the next lowest dose level if only 3 patients were treated previously at that dose.
≤1 of 6 at highest dose level below the maximally administered dose	This is generally the recommended phase 2 dose. At least 6 patients must be entered at the recommended phase 2 dose.

From NCI CTEP Phase 1 protocol template. Available at: http://ctep.cancer.gov/guidelines/templates.html.

the Veterinary Cooperative Oncology Group Common Terminology Criteria for Adverse Events (VCOG-CTCAE version 1.0) [14]. Grade IV is the cutoff most preferred for the DLT for bone marrow suppression in human trials, because these events are usually considered manageable and transient [5,12,13]. The MTD is defined as the highest dose level in which no more than one of six dogs develops a DLT. Traditionally, a fixed-dose modified Fibonacci method of dose escalation is used, wherein the dose is escalated 100%, 67%, 50%, 40%, and then 33% of the previous dose as the cohorts increase. Similar to starting at too low a dose, if the escalations are too conservative, more patients receive a suboptimal dose; however, if the escalations are too rapid, more patients are at risk for significant toxicity and the accuracy of the MTD is poor.

Alternative "accelerated titration" dose escalation strategies have been suggested [5,12,13]. These include (1) two-stage designs, wherein single-patient cohorts are used initially and dose is increased by a factor of 2 until a grade II toxicity occurs, and the second stage then involves more traditional three-patient cohorts and acceleration strategies; (2) within-patient escalation, wherein the same patient gets a higher dose on subsequent treatments until a DLT is observed (this may mask cumulative toxicity, however); (3) escalations based on PK parameters; (4) escalations based on target modification (if known); and (5) continuous reassessment methods using Bayesian methods (see subsequent section on Bayesian methods). In the end, it is always a trade-off of risk versus benefit; however, rapid accelerations are less likely to deny efficacious dosing to someone with a fatal disease [12].

As previously stated, although the phase I MTD approach works well for cytotoxic chemotherapeutics, it may be irrelevant for molecularly targeted drugs, and phase I trials designed to determine the BOD may be more relevant for so-called "static" agents. Trials evaluating the BOD need validated assays that measure target effect in serial tumor samples or some surrogate tissue or fluid that documents activity at the molecular level. One example would be measuring histone deacetylation in tumor tissue or surrogate peripheral blood mononuclear cells after the use of a histone deacetylase inhibitor, a promising new class of anticancer drugs (Fig. 2).

The author's group has been involved in several phase I trials in veterinary patients ranging from development of novel drugs to novel drug formulations and novel drug delivery systems [15–21]. For example, in a phase I trial in pet dogs, the DLT for liposomal doxorubicin was found to be a cutaneous toxicity (Fig. 3; palmar plantar erythrodysesthesia [PPES]) rather than hematologic or cardiac toxicity normally observed with nonliposomal doxorubicin [20]. In another phase I trial involving novel inhalational chemotherapeutics, data generated in pet dogs informed subsequent phase I trials in people with lung cancer (Fig. 4) [21,22].

Phase II Trials (Activity/Efficacy Trials)

Several good reviews have outlined phase II trial design [5,23–26]. The primary goal of phase II trials is, using the MTD established in phase I, to identify the clinical or biologic activity in defined patient populations (eg, tumors with

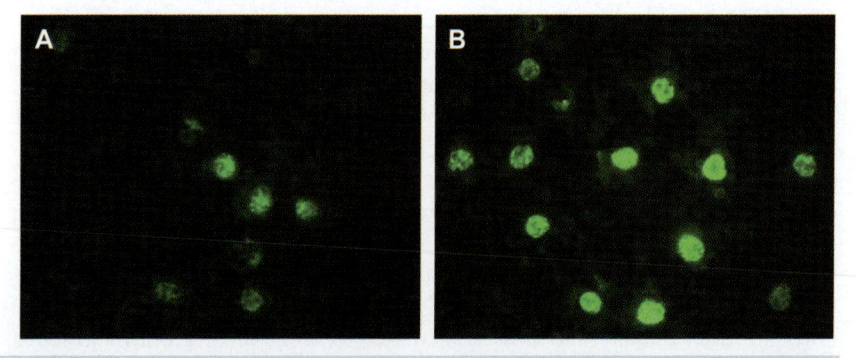

Fig. 2. Histone acetylation levels in peripheral blood mononuclear cells (PBMCs) before (A) and after (B) treatment of a dog with a histone deacetylase inhibitor that induces hyperacetylation. The degree of acetylation is measured by fluorescence microscopy using antiacetylated histone H3 polyclonal antisera. Such assays of surrogate tissues may be predictive of effects within the tumor. (*Courtesy of* D. Tham, VMD, Fort Collins, CO.)

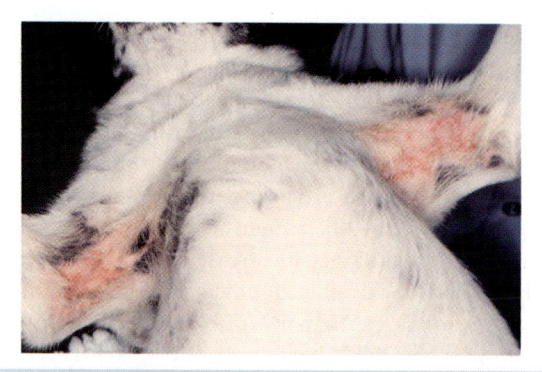

Fig. 3. Cutaneous toxicity involving the skin of the axilla in a dog after treatment with liposome-encapsulated doxorubicin (LED). This was determined to be the DLT in a phase I trial in pet dogs with cancer.

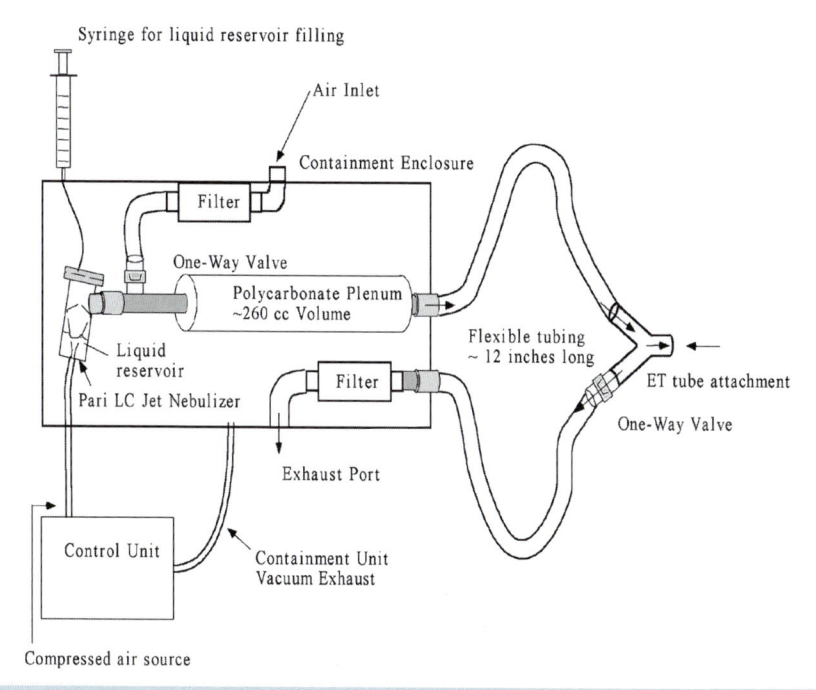

Fig. 4. Schematic diagram of the device used for phase I investigation of inhalational chemotherapy in pet dogs that had cancer. Results of this phase I trial in dogs subsequently informed phase I development in people who had lung cancer. (*From* Hershey AE, Kurzman ID, Bohling C, et al. Inhalation chemotherapy for macroscopic primary or metastatic lung tumors: proof of principle in a companion animal model. Clin Canc Res 1999;5:2655; with permission.)

a particular histology, tumors with a particular molecular target) and inform the decision to embark on a larger pivotal phase III trial. Other end points are summarized in Table 1. The traditional phase II design (phase IIA), the single-arm, open-label, phase II trial, is a nonrandomized nonblind activity assessment of a novel drug or therapeutic modality that lacks a control group or uses historical controls, which are prone to bias (selection, population drift, and stage migration bias) [25–28]. Simplistically, at least 9 patients with the same histology or molecular target are treated with the investigational drug to test the null hypothesis of insufficient efficacy [23]. Assuming the likelihood of spontaneous regression is less than 5% and expecting at least a 25% response rate for the agent to be clinically useful, with a $P \leq .05$ (type I [α] error; false positive) and a power of 0.8 (type II [β] error; false negative), if no responses are observed after nine cases, the study ends. If a response is noted in one of the cases, the accrual is increased to 31 patients to get an accurate response rate. If you expect a less sizable response rate, (eg, 5%–20%), the initial accrual number must be increased [25]. Some have opined that the leading cause of drug failure in later phase development is our overdependence on these unpredictable single-arm, uncontrolled, phase II trials in oncology and that, as such, they should be avoided to ensure phase III trial resources are not wasted because of the results of poorly designed phase II trials [24]. It used to be considered that the consequence of type I error (false positive) was less deleterious than that of type II error (false negative), because false-positive trials are likely to be repeated, whereas false-negative trials would result in the abandonment of a potentially active treatment. In today's environment, however, with an abundance of novel drugs to be evaluated, false-positive results are just as serious because they tie up patient and financial resources. With this in mind, the ideal phase II design would be randomized, blind, and controlled; modifications of this type applied to standard phase II design are discussed subsequently (controlled phase II trials).

End points of activity/efficacy
Because the primary goal of phase II trials is assessment of activity/efficacy, the end points used to evaluate response are critical to the design. With traditional cytotoxic chemotherapeutics, response criteria are fairly straightforward, because size or volume is used to assess response according to several published methodologies (eg, Response Evaluation Criteria in Solid Tumors [RECIST], World Health Organization [WHO]; Table 3) [29,30]. It is readily evident that such criteria may not be appropriate for the newer molecular targeting agents that are more likely to be cytostatic than cytotoxic and result in stabilization of disease rather than in measurable regression, however. In such cases, temporal measures, such as progression-free survival (PFS) or time to progression (TTP), would seem more appropriate end points; however, these often take too long to mature for timely phase II trials. Alternatively, an adequate compromise could be progression-free rate (PFR) at predetermined time points. Other end points for targeted agents could be a validated surrogate biomarker

Table 3
Definition of best response according to WHO or RECIST criteria

Best response	WHO change in sum of products	RECIST change in sums longest diameters
CR	Disappearance; confirmed at 4 weeks[a]	Disappearance; confirmed at 4 weeks[a]
PR	50% decrease; confirmed at 4 weeks[a]	30% decrease; confirmed at 4 weeks[a]
SD	Neither PR nor PD criteria met	Neither PR nor PD criteria met
PD	25% increase; no CR, PR, or SD documented before increased disease	20% increase; no CR, PR, or SD documented before increased disease

Abbreviations: CR, complete response; PD, progressive disease; PR, partial response; SD, stable disease.; RECIST, Response Evaluation Criteria in Solid Tumors; SD, stable disease; WHO, World Health Organization.
[a] This can vary.
From Therasse P, Arbuck SG, Eisenhauer EA, et al. New guidelines to evaluate the response to treatment in solid tumors. JNCI 2000;92(3):214; with permission.

or measure of a molecular effect, such as dephosphorylation of a growth factor receptor, changes in microvascular density, or specific target modulation (eg, see Fig. 2), that is linked to clinical outcome [26]. Secondary end points that can be evaluated in phase II trials are quality-of-life assessments, comparative cost of therapy, days of hospitalization, and toxicity, for example.

Importantly, phase II trials also serve to expand our knowledge of the cumulative or long-term toxicities of new agents that may not be observed in short-term phase I trials designed only to elucidate acute toxicity. An example of this in the veterinary literature involved a combined phase I/II trial simultaneously investigating the safety of liposome-encapsulated doxorubicin (LED) in cats while comparing its activity with native doxorubicin in cats with vaccine-associated sarcomas [31]. Unexpectedly, the MTD established for LED in the acute phase I component of the trial was found to result in delayed and dose-limiting nephrotoxicity after long-term follow-up in the phase II component of the trial (Fig. 5).

Controlled phase II trials
Sometimes referred to as phase IIB trials, these tend to be controlled, blind, and randomized investigations of two or more novel regimens that identify promising agents to send to phase III for additional evaluation. Regarding the ethics of control groups, placebo controls are generally not used in human clinical trials in the United States. Placebo controls or historical controls have been used in veterinary clinical trials if no standard of care exists or if the historical outcome for a particular tumor type is well documented and consistent. Examples of historical control trials in the veterinary literature often include cancer histologies with rapid and likely terminal progression (eg, advanced stage oral melanoma, stage II hemangiosarcoma) [32,33]. Randomized phase II trials can be as

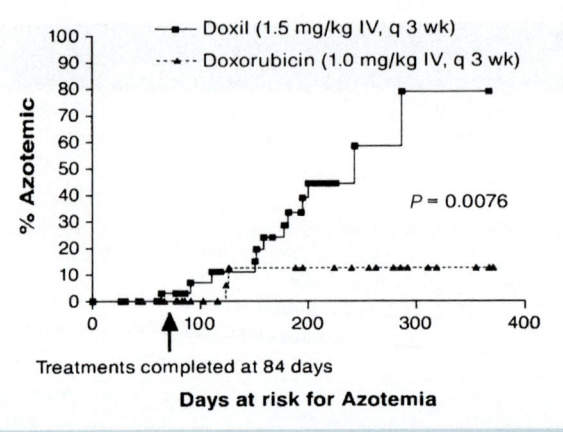

Fig. 5. A Kaplan-Meier curve comparing the probability of developing azotemia after the use of LED (Doxil) versus native doxorubicin in cats with vaccine-associated sarcoma [31]. This delayed toxicity was not observed in the phase I trial of Doxil and illustrates the limitations of the short-term nature of the design.

simple as randomizing standard of care plus or minus the addition of a new drug. More complicated trials can randomize subjects into multiple treatment arms or schedules with only enough power to make "inferences" as to which is the best drug to take forward into phase III, so-called "pick-the-winner" trials [25]. Although they often do not have enough power for direct comparison like a phase III trial would have, they may use a less rigorous statistical assessment, such as setting the P value at 10% and using one-tailed analysis. An example of a randomized phase II trial in veterinary medicine was mentioned previously and involved a randomized comparison of activity between LED and doxorubicin; neither agent had previously been the subject of a phase II activity trial in cats with vaccine-associated sarcoma [31]. A "winner" was not picked with respect to response activity in the macroscopic setting (44% response rate with LED versus 33% with doxorubicin; $P = .722$) or based on the temporal measurement of disease-free interval in the microscopic disease setting (Fig. 6). A clear winner (doxorubicin) was picked, however, when the secondary end points of cost and safety were factored in. Another randomized phase II trial that the author's group performed with LED involved pet dogs with non-Hodgkin's lymphoma (NHL) randomized to receive LED with pyridoxine or without pyridoxine [34]. The purpose of this phase II trial was to document activity in the NHL histology based on an MTD established in a previous phase I trial and, simultaneously, to determine if the addition of pyridoxine would diminish the DLT (PPES) also characterized in the earlier study [20]. Both objectives were met in that LED was found to be active for this histology (>70% objective response rate) and pyridoxine delayed and diminished the degree of PPES, allowing higher cumulative doses to be delivered (Fig. 7). Further examples of modified phase II trials, including seamless phase II/III trials,

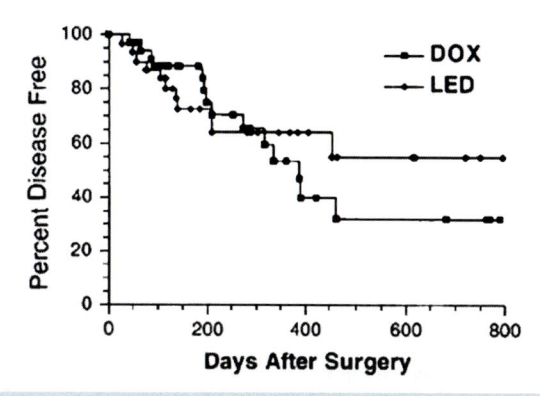

Fig. 6. Kaplan-Meier curve comparing the disease-free interval probability in cats treated with LED or native doxorubicin (DOX) generated in a phase II trial in cats with vaccine-associated sarcoma. (*From* Poirier VJ, Kurzman ID, Thamm DK, et al. LED (Doxil R) and doxorubicin in the treatment of vaccine-associated sarcoma in cats. J Vet Intern Med 2002;16:728; with permission.)

randomized discontinuation trials (RDTs), Bayesian continuous reassessment designs, and combinations are discussed in a subsequent section.

Phase III Trials (Comparative/Confirming Trials)

It has been suggested that if phase II trials are "learning" trials, phase III trials are "confirming" trials [8,26,35]. These larger, randomized, blind controlled

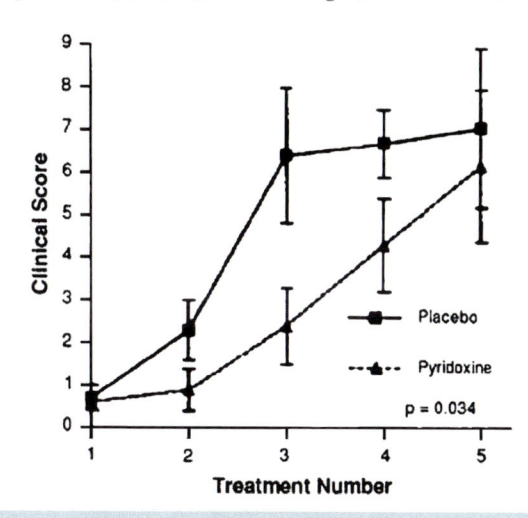

Fig. 7. Results of a randomized phase II trial performed with LED in pet dogs with NHL randomized to receive pyridoxine or placebo [34]. Pyridoxine delayed and diminished the degree of PPES, allowing higher cumulative doses of chemotherapy to be delivered. (*From* Vail DM, Chun R, Thamm DH, et al. Efficacy of pyridoxine to ameliorate the cutaneous toxicity associated with doxorubicin containing pegylated (stealth) liposomes: a randomized, double-blind clinical trial using a canine model. Clin Cancer Res 1998;4:1569; with permission.)

trials have the goal of comparing a new drug or combination with therapy regarded as the standard of care. They are often performed by large cooperative groups, which ensures greater case accrual. They are not common in veterinary medicine because of their size and expense. One example involving the multicenter approach would be the randomized comparison of liposome-encapsulated cisplatin (SPI-77) versus standard-of-care carboplatin in dogs with appendicular osteosarcoma [36] No difference was observed between treatment groups (Fig. 8), and SPI-77 did not show an activity advantage, despite allowing five times the MTD of native cisplatin to be delivered in a liposome-encapsulated form.

Phase IV Trials (Postmarket Trials)

Once a drug has been granted a license for a specific label use by the appropriate regulatory body (eg, Federal Drug Administration [FDA]), postmarket phase IV trials may be performed to gain more information on adverse events, safety, long-term risks, and benefits. Essentially, phase IV trials investigate the drug more widely than in the clinical trials used for licensure. They often involve treatment of special populations (eg, the elderly, children, individuals with renal or hepatic dysfunction) [5]. The body of data on PK generated from licensure trials is used to inform decisions on dose in these special populations.

MODIFICATIONS/ALTERNATIVES TO STANDARD CLINICAL TRIAL DESIGNS

Comments on Randomization

Randomization is the assignment of subjects into treatment groups based on chance-governed mechanisms, such as the flip of a coin, roll of the dice,

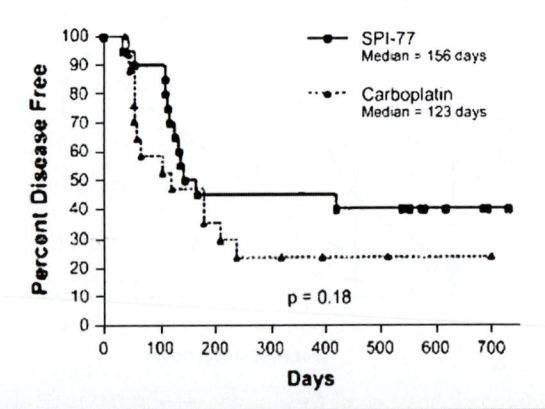

Fig. 8. Kaplan-Meier curve comparing the disease-free interval probability in dogs treated with SPI-77 or carboplatin generated in a phase III trial in pet dogs with osteosarcoma. (*From* Vail DM, ID Kurzman, PA Glawe, et al. Stealth liposomal cisplatin versus carboplatin as adjuvant therapy for spontaneously arising osteosarcoma in the dog: a randomized multicenter clinical trial. Cancer Chemother Pharmacol 2002;50:134; with permission.)

randomization tables, or computer programs. Each subject has an equal chance of being assigned to one treatment or the other. This is done to distribute equally known and, in particular, unknown factors that may affect outcome and to limit conscious and unconscious bias [35]. If the sample size is large enough, randomization is usually successful.

Regarding factors that are well known to affect outcome, a more specific form of randomization, stratification, can be used to ensure an equal distribution of patients with these factors within the treatment groups [37]. The classic example in veterinary cancer trials would be stratification by immunophenotype in dogs with NHL to ensure equal numbers of the poorly responding T-cell immunophenotype in the various treatment arms.

Unbalanced randomization schemes have also been proposed that allocate more subjects into one treatment group in an attempt to enhance the ethical palatability of some trials or to decrease the cost of trials; however, unbalanced randomization remains controversial [38,39].

The timing of randomization is also important. It is usually best to randomize as late as possible, because once randomization has occurred, subsequent analysis should be reported on an intention-to-treat basis rather than on a treatment-received basis [40,41]. All subjects should be included in the analysis regardless of whether they received all the prescribed treatments or not. This minimizes bias based on temporal issues or treatment toxicity. An example to illustrate this in veterinary oncology involves a presentation some years ago at an annual meeting that compared dogs with osteosarcoma receiving four doses of cisplatin after amputation with dogs receiving two doses of cisplatin. The conclusion, after treatment-received analysis, was that dogs receiving four doses lived longer. Because dogs that were scheduled to receive four treatments but did not because of early metastasis were excluded in the analysis, the four-treatment group data were biased to a positive result, because those dogs destined to metastasize early were removed, no matter how many treatments they would have received. That being said, it is acceptable to present treatment-received and intention-to-treat analyses in trial reports to discuss how loss to follow-up or treatment withdrawal may affect the conclusions. There are a few situations in which randomized patients can be removed from analysis, such as ineligible patients that are mistakenly randomized or those that are prematurely randomized but do not receive any intervention [40,41].

Phase 0 Trials

Recently the US FDA developed guidelines for exploratory investigational new drug studies, sometimes referred to as phase 0 trials [11,42]. These trials are exploratory clinical trials conducted before traditional dose escalation and safety studies are performed. They are designed to bridge the gap between preclinical and first-in-species phase I trials, help to make go/no go decisions, and provide a platform to establish the feasibility of assays for target modulation in samples from the target species [11]. In these short (usually 7 days or less) trials, small amounts of the drug (ie, 1% of the anticipated pharmacologically active dose: "homeopathic" or "microdose") are given to patients to establish whether the agent behaves in the target species as would be anticipated from preclinical studies. Therefore, these are intended for drugs that have a defined (understood) mechanism of action and for which investigators have some measurement (eg, biologic, pharmacologic, through bioimaging) that can determine whether the drug in question is hitting a target and having a desired effect—obviously a rare situation in the drug development realm [42]. Because such small amounts of drugs are used, these trials fit well with the needs of academic laboratories and small companies that want to evaluate the potential of the drug before scale-up to large production quantities. They are not intended to establish therapeutic intent or to define an MTD. The objectives of phase 0 trials include (1) determining if the agent has the correct PK/pharmacodynamics (PD) to be a contender (ie, does it enter the blood stream, does it interact with a key enzyme); (2) determining if the mechanism of action can be observed (ie, is an enzyme system intact and measurable in the target species); (3) possibly characterizing further the mechanism of action; (4) determining, validating, and refining a biomarker or imaging assay; (5) studying the effect of the drug in tumor samples or other surrogate tissues (and establishing standard operating procedures for tissue acquisition and handling); and (6) selecting the "lead agent" from a group of drugs.

The major theoretic advantages of phase 0 trials are that fewer preclinical (nontarget species) data are required than in a traditional phase I trial, only small batches of drug are necessary, the likelihood of an adverse event is low, and they are limited to a small number of subjects over a short period of time. The theoretic disadvantages of phase 0 trials are that we often do not know as much about target effects as we think, low-dose PK/PD may not recapitulate high-dose effects, they involve an extra development step, they may decrease the pool of patients eligible for phase I through III trials, and the nontherapeutic dose is not attractive to subjects (or their owners in the case of companion animals). Obviously, there are some ethical concerns surrounding phase 0 studies, because no therapeutic benefit is possible from subpharmacoactive drug quantities. It has thus been suggested that the best candidates for entry into phase 0 trials are patients having stable disease who do not have clinical signs requiring immediate therapy and who are not likely to progress in the 1 to 2 weeks they are ineligible for alternate therapy [11]. Ethical concerns could be lessened by allowing phase 0 participants to be eligible for future clinical trials and, indeed, offering them first crack at the phase I trial of the agent they are currently involved in with a phase 0 trial.

The author is unaware of any phase 0 trials being conducted in veterinary oncology. An example from the human oncology literature illustrating the potential utility of phase 0 trials concerns the development profile of metalloproteinase inhibitors. Despite a lack of observed effects on PD markers in early-phase trials, these agents proceeded to phase III trials in human beings (and phase II trials in dogs), in which they have generally failed, thereby squandering valuable resources and subjects.

Adaptive Trial Designs and Stopping Rules
Adaptive trial designs allow investigators to modify trials while they are ongoing based on data generated thus far and, in some cases, taking into account data generated in other trials or past trials.

Stopping rules
Stopping rules, rules that terminate a clinical trial earlier than originally projected or within a predetermined adaptive trial design, can be applied to randomized phase II or phase III trials. Several methods and variations have been extensively reviewed [8,26,43–45]. Stopping rules are designed to protect treatment subjects from unsafe drugs, to hasten the general availability of superior drugs as soon as sufficient evidence has been collected, and to help ensure the transfer of resources and patients to alternative trials. Trials are stopped for three reasons: the investigational treatment is clearly better than the control, the investigational treatment is clearly worse than the control (less activity or more toxicity), or the investigation's therapy is not likely to be better (so-called "stopping for futility" or "futility analysis"). The methods by which stopping rules are applied usually involve some type of interim analysis that looks at the data (by a blinded individual) generated so far and makes a determination based on predetermined rules. The interim data are often analyzed for conditional power, which is the probability of the final study result demonstrating statistical significance in the primary efficacy end point, conditional on the current data observed so far and a specific assumption about the pattern of the data to be observed in the remainder of the study [44,45]. If a study is designed up front to involve conditional power calculations of interim data, the rules for early termination are sometimes referred to as stochastic curtailing.

Bayesian (Continuous Learning) Adaptive Designs
Adaptive trial designs can be used not only to stop trials early but to adapt trials with respect to changing the randomization weight to better performing treatment arms, adding new treatment arms, dropping poorly performing arms, or extending accrual beyond the original target when more information is needed. With the availability of advance computational techniques, a new statistical methodology, the Bayesian approach, was developed that makes statistical inferences that focus on the probability that a hypothesis is true given the available evidence [46–51]. Traditionally, a frequentist approach to statistics is applied to clinical trials in which parameters are fixed and not subject to future probabilities and are inflexible. In contrast, Bayesian trials use available patient outcome information, including biomarkers that accumulate data related to outcome (if available and validated) and even historical information or results from other relevant trials. The Bayesian approach uses this information to adapt the current trial design continually based on newly informed probabilities. Bayesian designs are intrinsically adaptive and data driven, which allows inferences to depend less on the original study design [26]. Bayesian approaches can be incorporated into the trial at the beginning or can be used to monitor clinical trials originally designed with frequentist statistical methods.

An example that illustrates the utility of the Bayesian approach involves interim analysis applied to a randomized phase II trial of neoadjuvant epidermal growth factor receptor 2-positive breast cancer [52]. In this trial initially designed to enter 164 patients (based on the frequentist approach to power), a Bayesian approach was used to perform an interim analysis after 34 patients were enrolled; 67% of patients in the investigational treatment arm experienced complete responses compared with 25% in the standard treatment arm. The Bayesian predictive probability of statistical significance if 164 patients were accrued, based on the data available from these 34 patients, was calculated to be 95%, and the trial was stopped and the drug moved to phase III early.

Randomized Discontinuation Trials

This relatively new phase II design was proposed for evaluating the efficacy of newer targeted agents that are thought to have disease-stabilizing activity (cytostatic) in contrast to more traditional cytotoxic chemotherapeutics. Several reviews of this trial design are recommended [53–55]. Trials that evaluated growth-inhibiting agents in tumors with a variable natural history seem ideally suited for RDTs, because the "no treatment effect" is hard to control for in these cases. In essence, these trials serve to enrich (see later section) and homogenize for those patients likely to benefit from the static agent. RDTs involve a two-stage trial design (Fig. 9), wherein the first stage involves a "run-in" phase in which all patients receive the cytostatic agent under investigation. At the end of the run-in phase, assessment of disease response is made. If a response is noted, the subject continues on with the investigational drug, whereas if progression (or excess toxicity) is noted, the subject is removed from trial and allowed to receive alternative treatment. Those patients who meet stable disease criteria enter the second stage of the RDT and are randomized to continue

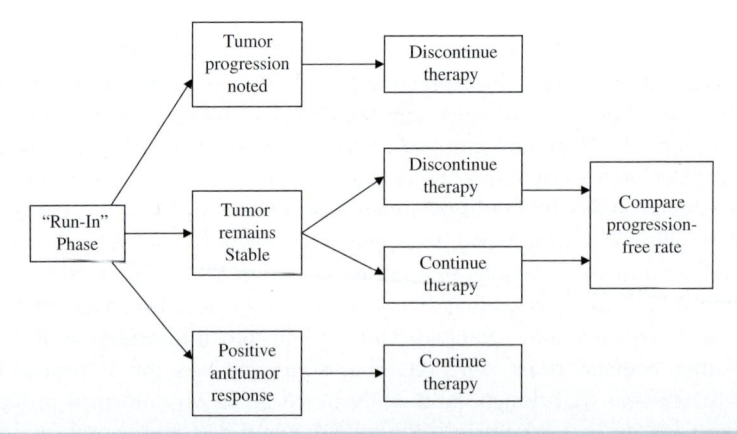

Fig. 9. Generalized schema for an RDT design. (*Adapted from* Stadler WM. The randomized discontinuation trial: a phase II design to assess growth-inhibitory agents. Mol Cancer Ther 2007;6(4):1182; with permission.)

on with the investigational drug or placebo (the discontinuation arm). Then, at predetermined times, follow-up determinations are made. End points in stage 2 of the trial at these follow-up intervals are "stable or better" versus "progression," that is, PFR. Time-to-event measures could be applied as well (eg, TTP), although this takes more time to complete. If a subject progresses in the second stage, the code can be broken, and if that subject is in the placebo group, the investigational drug can be reinstituted. Therefore, there are two ways for RDTs to be stopped: there are a substantial number of objective responses noted in the run-in phase, making a second stage unnecessary, or the number of subjects progressing in the second stage differs statistically between the treatment and placebo groups.

It becomes intuitive that the length of the run-in phase is critical to RDTs, because if it is too long, some initially responding patients progress during the late stage of the run-in and are missed (therefore increasing subject numbers); if it is too short, insufficient enrichment occurs (not enough time for nonresponders to progress) and the randomization might as well have been done at the outset. Therefore, it pays to have some preliminary ideas as to the natural history of the disease.

The two major advantages of RDTs are that all subjects receive the drug up front such that every patient is given a chance to respond to the drug (something that is popular with patients [or companion animal owners]) and enrichment of likely responders may increase power and decrease subject numbers. Potential disadvantages of RDTs include the ethics of discontinuation (but the design can allow reinstitution), the potential for a carry-over effect of the drug after discontinuation (unlikely for most targeted agents), and failure to detect short duration activity (but this would likely be a clinically irrelevant duration anyway). RDTs can be improved by combining other modifications of clinical trials, such as interim analysis and Bayesian analysis, and by using active controls.

For purposes of illustration, an RDT in veterinary medicine that the author has considered would be the investigation of a cytostatic agent in dogs with pulmonary metastatic osteosarcoma. All dogs would enter the run-in phase, receive the cytostatic drug for 4 weeks, and then be evaluated for response. From what we already know about the natural history of osteosarcoma in dogs, most (probably 80%) of dogs that did not receive treatment would progress in that period. Those that were stable at 4 weeks, however, would be randomized to drug continuation or discontinuation (placebo) and followed with monthly re-evaluations. This would ensure all dogs had a chance to respond to the drug and enrich the population likely to respond, and a positive result would be clinical response noted in the run-in phase or a statistical difference between groups in the second stage.

Phase Combinations
Several trials have combined the different phases (I/II/III) of clinical trials in the hope of streamlining and accelerating the drug development path as well as

decreasing the number of subjects needed by combining data from patients entered in earlier phases with those in later phases with regard to clinical outcome end points. These have been referred to as "parallel" or "seamless" phase I/II or phase II/III trials and have been reviewed [56–58]. For phase I/II combinations, after an initial period of dose escalation, patients are randomized to different admissible dose levels and Bayesian probabilities are used adaptively to assign patients into groups over time [56]. Doses with lower activity or unacceptable toxicity are eliminated, and those with higher activity are expanded. The combined trial is stopped when Bayesian probabilities for safety, activity, or futility hit prespecified boundaries. In phase II/III combinations, phase II learning is combined into phase III confirming [57,58]; that is, data generated for response in phase II continue into phase III. Treatment selection in phase III may be based on more short-term end points in the phase II portion (eg, surrogate biomarker, response rate), and all subjects (phases II and III) are then followed for more phase III–like confirmatory end points that take longer to mature (eg, overall survival, time to progression).

Enrichment

Enrichment involves an intent to select a population of subjects to randomize in a trial who are more homogeneous with respect to prognostic and, more importantly, predictive factors. Enrichment is used when the molecular target of the investigational drug is thought to be well known and there is some method to determine which subjects have tumors with the target and which do not. For example, if evaluating a novel compound that targets the epithelial growth factor receptor, immunohistochemistry could be performed on biopsy samples to ensure the presence of the receptor (Fig. 10), and only subjects with biopsies positive for the receptor would be eligible for inclusion in the trial. The classic

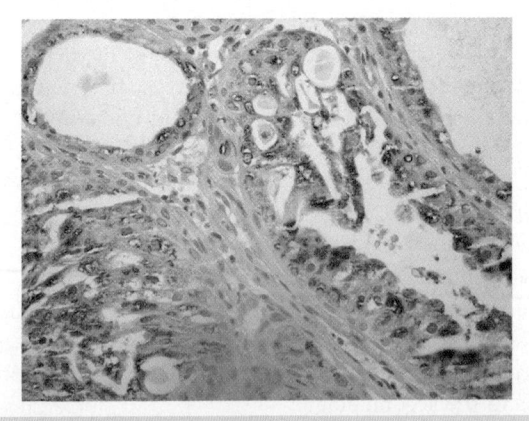

Fig. 10. Immunohistochemistry (IHC) of a section of transitional cell carcinoma from a dog. Amber staining represents positive epithelial growth factor receptor (EGFR) expression. IHC could be used to enrich a population of dogs for trials involving agents that target the EFGR pathway.

example cited to illustrate the power of enrichment is the seminal trial evaluating trastuzumab (*Her-2* monoclonal antibody) therapy combined with chemotherapy in women with breast cancer [59]. In this trial, 469 patients enriched for *Her-2*–expressing tumors were needed to show a statistical advantage with combination treatment (1-year overall survival of 78% versus 67%). It was estimated statistically that approximately 23,586 patients would have been required to show a similar difference in a population that was not enriched. One must be careful with enrichment, however, because many of the drugs we think of as specifically targeted actually have other targets that we are unaware of (so-called "dirty drugs" that have "off-target" effects) and we could miss a population of responders if we enriched only for what is know. An example would be evaluating tumors for responsiveness to imatinib, which is now known to inhibit 3 tyrosine kinase growth factor pathways (*Kit*, platelet-derived growth factor [PDGF], and Bcr-Abl) [60]. If we initially thought that imatinib only had activity against *Kit*-expressing tumors and enriched for them alone, patients with PDGF- and *Bcr-Abl*–driven tumors would be excluded from the study and potential responders would be lost.

Noninferiority Trials

Rather than demonstrating that a new drug is superior to standard of care, it is sometimes desirable to show that a drug is not inferior [61]. For example, a competing pharmaceutical company may wish to market a "me-too" drug of the same family that the company believes is as effective but has better PK parameters or a better safety profile, or one may wish to show that the addition of a drug that alleviates toxicity in a standard protocol does not also decrease the anticancer effects of the active agent. These are noninferiority trials. An example in the veterinary literature would be the previously mentioned pyridoxine/liposomal doxorubicin trial in which dogs were randomized to receive liposomal doxorubicin/placebo versus liposomal doxorubicin/pyridoxine [34]. In addition to determining that pyridoxine helped prevent the DLT of liposomal doxorubicin (PPES), an analysis was performed to ensure that activity (remission duration) was not adversely affected. These trials tend to be expensive with large numbers of subjects, because the definition of "inferior" must be predetermined and power must be sufficient to prove a negative result.

Crossover Trials

Crossover trials are a modification of a phase II or III trial in which subjects are randomized to receive one treatment arm or the other and then, after a certain trial period, enter a no-treatment washout phase (Fig. 11). After washout, they then are crossed over to receive the other treatment. Response end points are collected during both treatment phases and compared. This design increases the robustness of power, because patients serve as their own controls; therefore, paired data analysis can be used. Nevertheless, it is intuitive that this design is only well suited for chronic diseases that progress slowly (eg, arthritis, hypertension, diabetes, urinary incontinence) and for drugs that do not have a long carryover effect (longer than the washout period). They are rarely

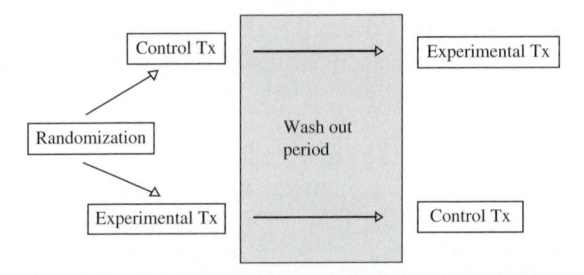

Fig. 11. Generalized schema for a crossover trial design. Tx, treatment.

used for cancer therapy trials because of the progressive nature of these diseases.

Informed Consent

The fact that the discussion of this component of clinical trials is at the end should not be construed to trivialize it. Rather, this is a critical component of any trial; as investigators, we are ethically bound to ensure that our clients are informed of the design complexity, the risks (known and unknown), and the benefits (or lack thereof) of any trial they may be considering for their companion animal before entry. Several reviews have addressed these concerns in physician-based oncology [62–64]. The 14 components of consent found on the Morris Animal Foundations web site [65] are recommended by the author to be included in any clinical trial consent form (Box 1).

> **Box 1: Suggested "elements of consent" to include in informed client consent documents**
>
> 1. Purpose of research
> 2. Expected duration of participation
> 3. Description of procedures
> 4. Possible discomforts and risks
> 5. Possible benefits
> 6. Alternative treatment (or alternative to participation)
> 7. Extent of confidentiality of records
> 8. Compensation or therapy for injuries
> 9. Contact person for the study
> 10. Voluntary participation and right to withdraw
> 11. Termination of participation by the principal investigator
> 12. Unforeseen risks
> 13. Financial obligations
> 14. Hospital review committee contact person
>
> *Courtesy of* Morris Animal Foundation, Englewood, CO; with permission.

SUMMARY

The application of rigorously controlled clinical trials is a relatively new concept in veterinary oncology, and clinical trial design has been an afterthought in most veterinary medical curricula. A working understanding of trial design and implementation is important for trial investigators and the clinicians who read trial reports to recognize fully the strengths and weaknesses of the reported data. This is a necessary prerequisite to make appropriate conclusions and ultimately advance the standard of care in clinical practice. Although much of the current standard of care in veterinary oncology is based on retrospective studies or transference from the human literature, a new era of clinical trial awareness brought on by new consortia and cooperative investigative groups is beginning to change this limitation. The use of controlled, randomized, blind multicenter trials testing new cytotoxics and cytostatic agents is now becoming the norm rather than the exception. Ultimately, advanced clinical trial design applied to companion animal populations should advance veterinary-based practice and inform future human clinical trials that may follow.

APPENDIX I (GLOSSARY OF TERMS)

Active controls are subjects in the control group who receive an active agent rather than a placebo.

Adaptive trial designs allow modifications to occur while trials are ongoing based on data generated thus far and, in some cases, taking into account data generated in other trials or past trials.

Bayesian approach to statistical analysis is focused on the probability that a hypothesis is true, given the available evidence. It represents the inverse of the more traditional frequentist approach.

Cohort study is a study in which patients who have a certain condition or receive a particular treatment are followed over time and compared with patients in another group who are not affected by the condition under investigation.

Conditional power is the probability of the final study result demonstrating statistical significance in the primary efficacy end point, conditional on the current data observed so far and a specific assumption about the pattern of the data to be observed in the remainder of the study.

Enrichment is the intent to select a population of subjects for a clinical trial that is more homogeneous with respect to prognostic and, more importantly, predictive factors.

First-in-species trial is a phase I trial in which the investigational treatment is being used in that species for the first time.

Frequentist approach to statistical analysis is focused on the probability of results of a trial assuming that a particular hypothesis is true.

Futility analysis is a form of interim analysis seeking to determine if the continuation of a trial is futile with respect to rejecting the null hypothesis; that is, the investigation drug is not showing superior activity and is not likely to even with additional subject accrual.

Intention-to-treat analysis asserts that all randomized subjects are included in statistical analysis regardless of whether they received all the prescribed treatments or not.

Null hypothesis (H_0) is a hypothesis set up to be nullified or refuted to support an alternative hypothesis and is presumed to be true until statistical evidence indicates otherwise. With respect to clinical trials comparing two treatment groups, the null hypothesis assumes that no difference exists and the alternative hypothesis assumes that a difference does exist.

Phase 0 trials are exploratory clinical trials conducted before traditional dose escalation and safety studies are performed.

Phase I (dose-finding) trials are defined in Table 1.

Phase II (activity/efficacy) trials are defined in Table 1.

Phase III (comparative) trials are defined in Table 1.

Phase IV (postmarketing) trials are clinical trials performed after licensure that expand the populations exposed to the investigational therapy to specific groups (eg, elderly, pediatric, organ failure).

Prognostic factors identify patients at generally higher risk of developing recurrence or death as the result of a particular cancer.

Predictive factors identify patients who are more or less likely to benefit from a specific therapy.

Prospective clinical trials look forward in time and are designed to collect data regarding events that occur in the future.

Randomization is the assignment of subjects into treatment groups based on chance-governed mechanisms, such as the flip of a coin, roll of the dice, randomization tables, or computer programs.

Retrospective studies look backward in time and collect data regarding events that occurred in the past, for example, pulling records of cases of dogs that have died of hemangiosarcoma and "mining" the record for data.

Standard of care is the current consensus "gold standard" therapy for a particular patient having a similar tumor of a similar clinical stage.

Stochastic curtailing is the use of prespecified limitations that, if reached after conditional power calculations of interim data, terminate the clinical trial. It represents a type of stopping rule.

Stopping rules terminate a clinical trial after some interim analysis (planned or unplanned) because of superior activity, increased toxicity, or futility.

Stratification is a form of randomization in which subjects are first placed within similar strata (groups) based on known prognostic/predictive factors and then randomized so as to ensure an equal distribution of patients with these factors within each treatment group.

Type I (α) error occurs when the null hypothesis is rejected when it is, in fact, true. In other words, a difference is found when none exists (ie, a false-positive result). It is represented as a P value (eg, $P < 0.05$ means there is a 5% chance that the difference observed was attributable to type I error).

Type II (β) error occurs when the null hypothesis is accepted when it is, in fact, false. In other words, no difference was found when one actually exists (ie, a false-negative result). It is often stated in terms of power, wherein $1 - \beta =$ power (eg, if β is 0.2, power is 0.8 or there is an 80% chance that you are making the correct decision by accepting the null hypothesis).

Unbalanced randomization is a type of randomization in which more subjects are put on one treatment arm when there is a strong suggestion that it may prove superior (eg, 2 to 1 randomization results in twice as many subjects in one arm than in another).

References

[1] Mack GS. Clinical trials going to the dogs; canine program to study tumor treatment, biology. J Natl Cancer Inst 2006;98(3):161–2.
[2] Mack GS. Cancer researchers usher in dog days of medicine. Nat Med 2005;11(10): 1018.
[3] Khanna C, Lindblad-Toh K, Vail D, et al. The dog as a cancer model. Nat Biotechnol 2006;24(9):1065–6.
[4] Waters DJ, Wildasin K. Cancer clues from pet dogs. Sci Am 2006;295(6):94–101.
[5] Kummar S, Gutierrez M, Doroshow JH, et al. Drug development in oncology; classical cytotoxics and molecularly targeted agents. Br J Clin Pharmacol 2006;62(1):15–26.
[6] Kamb A, Wee S, Lengauer C. Why is cancer drug discovery so difficult. Nat Rev Drug Discov 2007;6(2):115–20.
[7] Kamb A. What's wrong with our cancer models? Nat Rev Drug Discov 2005;4(2):161–5.
[8] Whitehead J. Stopping clinical trials by design. Nat Rev Drug Discov 2004;3(11):973–7.
[9] Booth B, Glassman R, Ma P. Oncology trials. Nat Rev Drug Discov 2003;2(8):609–10.
[10] Von Hoff DD. There are no bad anticancer agents, only bad clinical trial designs: Twenty-First Richard and Hinda Rosenthal Foundation Award Lecture. Clin Cancer Res 1998;4: 1079–86.
[11] Kummar S, Kinders R, Rubinstien L, et al. Compressing drug development timelines in oncology using phase '0' trials. Nat Rev Cancer 2007;7(2):131–9.
[12] Potter DM. Phase I studies of chemotherapeutic agents in cancer patients: a review of the designs. J Biopharm Stat 2006;16(5):579–604.
[13] Acevedo PV, Toppmeyer DL, Rubin EH. Phase I trial design and methodology for anticancer drugs. In: Teicher BA, Andrews PA, editors. Anticancer drug development guide. 2nd edition. Totowa (NJ): Humana Press; 2004. p. 351–62.
[14] Vail DM. Veterinary Co-Operative Oncology Group—common terminology criteria for adverse events following chemotherapy or biological antineoplastic therapy in dogs and cats. Veterinary and Comparative Oncology 2004;2(4):194–213.
[15] Thamm DH, Kurzman ID, King I, et al. Systemic administration of an attenuated, tumor-targeting Salmonella typhimurium to dogs with spontaneous neoplasia: phase I evaluation. Clin Cancer Res 2005;11:4827–34.
[16] Poirier VJ, Burgess KE, Adams WM, et al. Toxicity, dose and efficacy of vinorelbine (Navelbine®) in dogs with spontaneous neoplasia. J Vet Intern Med 2004;18:536–9.
[17] Poirier VJ, Hershey AE, Burgess KE, et al. Efficacy and toxicity of paclitaxel (Taxol®) for the treatment of canine malignant tumors. J Vet Intern Med 2004;18:219–22.
[18] Khanna C, Vail DM. Targeting the lung: preclinical and comparative evaluation of anticancer aerosols in dogs with naturally occurring cancers. Curr Cancer Drug Targets 2003;3: 265–73.
[19] Thamm DH, MacEwen EG, Phillips BS, et al. Preclinical study of dolastatin-10 in dogs with spontaneous neoplasia. Cancer Chemother Pharmacol 2002;49:251–5.
[20] Vail DM, Kravis LD, Cooley AJ, et al. Preclinical trial of doxorubicin entrapped in sterically stabilized liposomes in dogs with spontaneously arising malignant tumors. Cancer Chemother Pharmacol 1997;39:410–6.
[21] Hershey AE, Kurzman ID, Bohling C, et al. Inhalation chemotherapy for macroscopic primary or metastatic lung tumors: proof of principle in a companion animal model. Clin Cancer Res 1999;5:2653–9.
[22] Otterson GA, Villalona-Calero MA, Sharma S, et al. Phase I study of inhaled doxorubicin for patients with metastatic tumors to the lungs. Clin Cancer Res 2007;13(4):1246–52.

[23] Simon R. Optimal two-stage designs for phase II clinical trial. Control Clin Trials 1989;10(1):1–10.
[24] Michaelis LC, Ratain MJ. Phase II trials published in 2002: a cross-specialty comparison showing significant design differences between oncology trials and other medical specialties. Clin Cancer Res 2007;13(8):2400–5.
[25] Gray R, Manola J, Saxman S, et al. Phase II clinical trial design: methods in translational research from the Genitourinary Committee at the Eastern Cooperative Oncology Group. Clin Cancer Res 2006;12(7):1966–9.
[26] Lee JJ, Feng L. Randomized phase II designs in cancer clinical trials: current status and future directions. J Clin Oncol 2005;23(19):4450–7.
[27] Gehan EA. The determination of the number of patients required in a preliminary and a follow-up trial of a new chemotherapeutic agent. J Chronic Dis 1961;13:346–53.
[28] Fleming TR. One sample multiple testing procedure for phase AII clinical trials. Biometrics 1982;38:143–51.
[29] Therasse P, Arbuck SG, Eisenhauer EA, et al. New guidelines to evaluate the response to treatment in solid tumors. J Natl Cancer Inst 2000;92(3):205–16.
[30] WHO handbook for reporting results of cancer treatment. Geneva (Switzerland): World Health Organizations Offset Publication No. 48; 1979.
[31] Poirier VJ, Kurzman ID, Thamm DK, et al. Liposome-encapsulated doxorubicin (Doxil R) and doxorubicin in the treatment of vaccine-associated sarcoma in cats. J Vet Intern Med 2002;16:726–31.
[32] Bergman PJ, McKnight J, Novosad A, et al. Long-term survival of dogs with advanced malignant melanoma after DNA vaccination with xenogeneic human tyrosinase. Clin Cancer Res 2003;9:1284–90.
[33] Alexander AN, Huelsmeyer MK, Mitzey M, et al. Development of an allogeneic whole-cell tumor vaccine expressing xenogeneic gp100 and its implementation in a phase II clinical trial in canine patients with malignant melanoma. Cancer Immunol Immunother 2006;55:433–42.
[34] Vail DM, Chun R, Thamm DH, et al. Efficacy of pyridoxine to ameliorate the cutaneous toxicity associated with doxorubicin containing pegylated (stealth) liposomes: a randomized, double-blind clinical trial using a canine model. Clin Cancer Res 1998;4:1567–71.
[35] Dagher RN, Pazdur R. The phase III clinical cancer trial. In: Teicher BA, Andrews PA, editors. Anticancer drug development guide. 2nd edition. Totowa (NJ): Humana Press; 2004. p. 401–10.
[36] Vail DM, Kurzman ID, Glawe PA, et al. Stealth liposomal cisplatin versus carboplatin as adjuvant therapy for spontaneously arising osteosarcoma in the dog: a randomized multicenter clinical trial. Cancer Chemother Pharmacol 2002;50:131–6.
[37] Friedman LM, Furberg CD, DeMets DL. The randomization process. In: Fundamentals of clinical trials. 2nd edition. Littleton (MA): PSG Publishing; 1985. p. 51–69.
[38] Edwards S, Braunholtz D. Can unequal be more fair? A response to Andrew Avins. J Med Ethics 2000;26:179–82. doi:10.1136/jme.26.3.179.
[39] Avins AL. Can unequal be more fair? Ethics, subject allocation, and randomised clinical trials. J Med Ethics 1998;24:401–8.
[40] Montori VM, Guyatt GH. Intention-to-treat principle. Can Med Assoc J 2001;165(10):1339–41.
[41] Fergusson D, Aaron SD, Guyatt G, et al. Post-randomization exclusion: the intention to treat principle and excluding patients from analysis. Br Med J 2002;325(7365):652–5.
[42] Twombly R. Slow start to phase 0 as researchers debate value. J Natl Cancer Inst 2006;98(12):804–6.
[43] Lee JJ, Lieberman R, Sloan JA, et al. Design considerations for efficient prostate cancer chemoprevention trials. Urology 2001;57(4 Suppl 1):206–12.
[44] Betensky RA. Conditional power calculations for early acceptance of H_o embedded in sequential tests. Stat Med 1997;16:465–77.

[45] Lachin JM. A review of methods for futility stopping based on conditional power. Stat Med 2004;24:2747–64.
[46] Berry DA. Bayesian clinical trials. Nat Rev Drug Discov 2006;5:27–36.
[47] Johns D, Andersen JS. Use of predictive probabilities in phase II and phase III clinical trials. J Biopharm Stat 1999;9:67–9.
[48] Berry DA, Eick SG. Adaptive assignment versus balanced randomization in clinical trials: a decision analysis. Stat Med 1995;14:231–46.
[49] Thall PF, Wathen JK, Bekele BN, et al. Hierarchical Bayesian approaches to phase II trials in diseases with multiple subtypes. Stat Med 2003;22:763–80.
[50] Inoue LY, Thall PF, Berry DA. Seamlessly expanding a randomized phase II trial to phase III. Biometrics 2002;58:823–31.
[51] Stallard N, Thall PF, Whitehead J. Decision theoretic designs for phase II clinical trials with multiple outcomes. Biometrics 1999;55:971–7.
[52] Buzdar AU, Ibrahim NK, Francis D, et al. Significantly higher pathologic complete remission rate after neoadjuvant therapy with trastuzumab, paclitaxel, and epirubicin chemotherapy; results of a randomized trial in human epidermal growth factor receptor 2-positive operable breast cancer. J Clin Oncol 2005;23(16):3676–85.
[53] Stadler WM. The randomized discontinuation trial: a phase II design to assess growth-inhibitory agents. Mol Cancer Ther 2007;6(4):1180–5.
[54] Stadler WM, Rosner G, Small E, et al. Successful implementation of the randomized discontinuation trial design: an application to the study of the putative antiangiogenic agent carboxyaminoimidazole in renal cell carcinoma—CALGB 69901. J Clin Oncol 2005;23(16):3726–32.
[55] Rosner GL, Stadler W, Ratain MJ. Randomized discontinuation design: application to cytostatic antineoplastic agents. J Clin Oncol 2002;20(22):4478–84.
[56] Huang X, Biswas S, Oki Y, et al. A parallel phase I/II clinical trial design for combination therapies. Biometrics 2006;1–8.
[57] Maca J. Adaptive seamless phase II/III designs—background, operational aspects and examples. Drug Inf J 2006;40(04):463–74.
[58] Bretz F, Schmidli H, Konig F, et al. Confirmatory seamless phase II/III clinical trials with hypothesis selection at interim: general concepts. Biom J 2006;48(4):623–34.
[59] Slamon DJ, Leyland-Jones B, Shak S, et al. Use of chemotherapy plus a monoclonal antibody against HER2 for metastatic breast cancer that overexpresses HER2. N Engl J Med 2001;344(11):783–92.
[60] Jones RL, Judson IR. The development and application of imatinib. Expert Opin Drug Saf 2005;4(2):183–91.
[61] Tsong Y, Chen WJ. Noninferiority testing beyond simple two-sample comparison. J Biopharm Stat 2007;17(2):289–308.
[62] Cox AC, Fallowfield LJ, Jenkins VA. Communication and informed consent in phase 1 trials: a review of the literature. Support Care Cancer 2006;14(4):303–9.
[63] Jayson G, Harris J. How participants in cancer trials are chosen: ethics and conflicting interests. Nat Rev Cancer 2006;6(4):330–6.
[64] Albrecht TL, Franks MM, Ruckdesche JC. Communication and informed consent. Curr Opin Oncol 2005;17(4):336–9.
[65] Morris Animal Foundations. Available at: www.morrisanimalfoundation.org/reports/grants/full_proposal/Established_Investigator_guidelines.pdf.

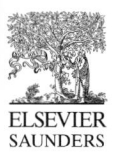

Advanced Imaging for Veterinary Cancer Patients

Amy K. LeBlanc, DVM[a,*], Gregory B. Daniel, DVM, MS[b]

[a]Department of Small Animal Clinical Sciences, College of Veterinary Medicine, University of Tennessee, C247 Veterinary Teaching Hospital, Knoxville, TN 37996-4544, USA
[b]Department of Small Animal Clinical Sciences, Virginia-Maryland Regional College of Veterinary Medicine, Virginia Polytechnic Institute and State University, Mail Code 0442, Blacksburg, VA 24061, USA

This article presents an update on the recent advances made in veterinary advanced imaging specifically with regard to cross-sectional modalities (CT and MRI) and nuclear medicine (positron emission tomography [PET] and PET/CT). A brief summary of technical improvements and a review of recent literature are included to provide an overview of the progress made in this important element of the practicing veterinary oncologist's repertoire. An in-depth summary of PET is also included to introduce the technical aspects and potential clinical and research applications of this novel imaging modality in veterinary medicine.

There is little debate on the importance of diagnostic imaging in veterinary oncologic practice. Radiography and ultrasonography are now commonplace; more advanced cross-sectional imaging modalities, such as CT or MRI, are becoming routinely available in private referral practices and academic centers alike. Veterinary oncologists now frequently rely on advanced imaging techniques for optimal patient staging and management. The past decade has seen a vast improvement in the collective experience and knowledge base pertaining to cross-sectional imaging studies, specifically CT and MRI, in veterinary patients.

Although CT and MRI provide high-resolution imaging, they are limited in their ability to detect neoplastic disease before significant anatomic alterations occur. PET is an important imaging technique commonly used in the diagnosis, staging, and management of neoplastic disease in human beings. With the recent advent of PET/CT fusion technology, the advantages of anatomic and functional imaging are realized in a single study. Potential applications of PET and PET/CT to clinical veterinary oncology are numerous and include diagnosis and initial staging of malignancy, assessment of response to therapy, and detection of recurrent disease after treatment. PET and PET/CT have many

*Corresponding author. E-mail address: aleblanc@utk.edu (A.K. LeBlanc).

applications as research tools in studying spontaneous cancer development in animals and aiding in novel radiotracer development.

CROSS-SECTIONAL IMAGING MODALITIES: CT AND MRI
CT
Technical advances

A CT scanner is an x-ray–producing machine that creates cross-sectional images of the body. The principles of image formation are similar to those of a conventional x-ray machine. The image formation is based on the magnitude of attenuation of the x-ray beam as it passes through the body. This differential absorption of the x-ray beam creates the various radiographic opacities (metal, bone, water, fat, and air) seen on the conventional radiograph. A CT image is also formed by attenuation of the x-ray beam by the various tissues; however, it is not limited to just the five basic radiographic opacities. Each picture element (voxel) of the CT image represents the magnitude of attenuation by that particular volume of tissue. The magnitude of attenuation is expressed as a normalized CT number or Hounsfield unit (HU). The attenuation coefficient for each voxel is normalized to the attenuation coefficient of distilled water. The range of HUs varies from -1000 (air) to $+3000$, with water having a value of 0. Availability of CT is increasing in academic and private practices.

Most human imaging centers have replaced later generation axial scanners with single or multislice spiral (helical) scanners. Traditional axial scanners rotate the x-ray tube around the patient for each image slice. After completion of tube rotation, the table moves the patient to the next position and the process is repeated in an expose-move-expose fashion. Spiral CT scanners move the patient through the gantry at a constant speed while the x-ray tube continuously rotates around the patient, making one long exposure through the anatomic area of interest. Spiral CT has become the method of choice for many newer clinical studies, providing good image quality with reasonably short acquisition times. A further increase in the table transport speed (eg, volume coverage speed) generally results in clinically unacceptable images, however. Further improvements in imaging speed are needed for many time-critical applications, such as pulmonary embolism studies, dual-phase liver studies, CT angiography, or neurologic and whole-body trauma.

In the early 1990s, a two-detector array scanner was introduced that could generate two image slices in the time previously required for one slice; this technology is currently referred to as multislice CT. Over the past 15 years, the number of slices acquired per tube rotation has increased dramatically, with 40- and 60-slice scanners found commonly in human imaging facilities. With the advent of multislice CT, the price of used and refurbished axial and single-slice spiral scanners has dropped into a range that is affordable for many veterinary practices. Today, there are veterinary imaging centers with high-quality later generation CT scanners that are capable of producing high-resolution axial images of veterinary patients.

The use of contrast media in CT studies improves the observed soft tissue contrast and helps to define neoplastic lesions and their extension into surrounding tissues better. Most imaging protocols call for the same image set to be acquired before and after intravenous administration of a nonionic iodinated contrast agent. The contrast may be administered as an intravenous bolus or as a constant rate infusion using a power injector if available. After contrast administration, a second set of images is acquired a few seconds after injection of the contrast bolus or during the time of contrast infusion. The contrast agent accumulates in highly vascular tissue or in tissues with increased vascular permeability. The margins of many neoplastic lesions appear more conspicuous after contrast administration. Because contrast-enhanced CT is useful for assessment of tumor vascularity and regional blood flow, this technique is applicable to quantitative studies of perfusion and permeability for investigation of angiogenesis and cellular hypoxia. Dynamic CT measurement of contrast medium "wash-in" kinetics was performed in a series of nine dogs with nasal tumors in an effort to assess tumor perfusion before and during radiation therapy, but no identifiable pattern of perfusion change was noted [1]. Contrast-enhanced CT was also used to assess perfusion and permeability of tumors in a xenograft rodent model system [2].

CT can also be used to assist in biopsy or fine-needle aspiration of suspected neoplastic lesions, with guided percutaneous biopsy techniques widely described in veterinary patients for tissue diagnosis of neoplasms located within the head, spine, thorax, abdomen, and bone [3,4]. CT-guided fine-needle aspiration and tissue-core biopsy were associated with high accuracy (95.7%) in the diagnosis of bone lesions (orbital, spinal, nasal, long bones, and bulla) in dogs and cats [5].

Clinical applications
Brain and spinal/paraspinal tumors. It is widely accepted that cross-sectional imaging is essential to the diagnosis of intracranial tumors, providing a high level of anatomic detail that cannot be gleaned from survey radiography because of superimposition of bony structures of the head. The first reports of cross-sectional imaging to characterize intracranial neoplasia in companion animals appear in the early 1980s using CT [6–8]. The first comprehensive study of canine brain tumors was published in 1984, describing the CT characteristics of various brain tumor histologic findings [9]. Since then, many studies have demonstrated the advantages and disadvantages of this modality for diagnosis of intracranial tumors. Some lesions may not be visible with CT because of poor differentiation from surrounding tissue, poor contrast enhancement, or diffuse distribution within the brain [10]. Lesions within the brain stem, adjacent to the petrous temporal bone, may be obscured by beam-hardening artifacts. These artifacts are attributable to computer miscalculations of the attenuation coefficient of tissue deep to high-density material, such as the bone at the base of the skull. Hypoattenuating streaks characteristic of beam hardening may prevent lesion detection in this area.

The common CT features of canine and feline intracranial tumors have been compiled from several references [11]. Most brain tumors are isoattenuating on CT (have the same density as normal brain) before contrast medium administration. Tumors that have relatively normal vasculature and are slowly growing with a lack of other noticeable pathologic findings, such as edema or falx shift, may go undetected on CT [11]. As discussed elsewhere in this article, MRI shows greater promise in characterization of neoplasia involving the central nervous system (CNS) because of superior anatomic detail, ability to resolve small tumors, and improved soft tissue contrast [11].

CT provides valuable information for guidance of surgical procedures and planning of radiotherapy for highly contrast-enhancing brain lesions, such as pituitary macroadenomas, meningiomas, and choroid plexus tumors [12]. CT can also be used for guidance of stereotactic brain biopsies using modified human systems with a high rate of diagnostic yield (>90%), with minimal postprocedural complications (epistaxis, altered neurologic status, and seizures) in most studied dogs, although rare postprocedural deaths were reported [13–16]. Traditional surgical management of brain tumors is becoming more common, largely because of increased availability of CT and MRI, along with advances in neurosurgical techniques [10].

External-beam radiation therapy can be used for intracranial lesions that cannot be managed surgically or as an adjuvant treatment to surgery or chemotherapy. CT images are routinely used to ensure accurate patient setup and positioning for definitive radiation therapy. Most computer-based treatment planning software can receive the digital imaging and communications in medicine image files imported from a CT scanner. A recent report described the utility of megavoltage CT (MVCT) images from a clinical helical tomotherapy system for setup verification purposes for veterinary patients undergoing definitive radiation therapy. The investigators found that MVCT images can be aligned with the routine planning CT images of the patient to allow proper patient positioning before treatment without skin markings [17]. Similarly, CT images were used in another study in concert with a fixed immobilization device to allow repeatable patient positioning for radiation treatment of head region tumors [18]. Radiosurgery using a stereotactic headframe to deliver a single dose (1000–1500 cGy) of radiation to three dogs with brain tumors was also reported with good outcome and no procedural complications [19].

CT can also be used to restage animals that have had surgery or radiotherapy as treatment for intracranial neoplasia to evaluate response to therapy or to investigate the cause of new or worsening neurologic signs. As discussed elsewhere in this article, PET and PET/CT may be more helpful than purely anatomic imaging because PET can differentiate between scar and metabolically active tumor cells that represent tumor recurrence after surgery or radiotherapy.

Application of CT for evaluation of spinal and nerve root tumors is also described. CT is useful in guiding diagnostic and therapeutic procedures for spinal tumors, because superimposition of surrounding bony structures precludes use of standard radiographic techniques for surgical or radiotherapy planning

[20–23]. In a recent study of 24 dogs with tumors of the brachial plexus and contributing nerve roots, no specific relation between tomographic appearance and histology could be defined [20].

Non-central nervous system head and neck neoplasia

Nasal tumors. Many reports describe the CT features of various intranasal disease processes and how the features of neoplastic disease differ from non-neoplastic processes [24–30]. Nasal CT greatly enhances the clinician's ability to diagnose and stage intranasal neoplasia. CT can identify optimal areas for rhinoscopy and biopsy to confirm the cause of the disease process in question. For dogs with intranasal neoplasia, CT provides an accurate assessment of tumor size, extent of disease within or outside the nasal cavity, and presence of bony destruction [25,26]. In addition, CT can assess regional lymph nodes to determine the likelihood of metastatic involvement based on size or contrast enhancement [12]. These variables can also be helpful in treatment planning and predicting the degree of normal tissue toxicity expected with definitive radiation therapy in this anatomic region.

For cats with intranasal disease, CT characteristics significantly associated with sinonasal neoplasia were unilateral lysis of the ethmoturbinates; dorsal, lateral, or ventral maxilla; or vomer bone; bilateral lysis of orbital lamina and collection of unilateral abnormal soft tissue or fluid within the sphenoid and frontal sinuses or retrobulbar space were also seen [30]. Another study of cats with sinonasal disease found that CT was not more sensitive than parallel radiographic studies at detecting nasal cavity abnormalities but was more sensitive in localizing these changes and determining the extent of disease [29].

Tumors of the skull and oral cavity. CT has become an important component of oral tumor staging, because invasion into the mandible or maxilla and extension of the tumor into the nasal cavity, caudal pharynx, and orbit can be defined. Evidence of regional lymph node metastasis (eg, nodal enlargement, contrast enhancement) can also be gleaned with CT. Many studies of intraoral neoplasia demonstrate the importance of tumor stage and presence or absence of bony involvement as prognostic factors for remission and survival; therefore, CT is an invaluable part of intraoral tumor staging. Similarly, tumors involving the skull can easily be imaged with CT for staging and treatment planning purposes [31–35]. As expected, a bone window is best in this setting to accentuate tumor-associated bone destruction [32].

Intrathoracic neoplasia

Primary lung tumors. Detection of pulmonary tumors is easily accomplished with plain radiographs that provide a global view of the thorax. Accurate assessment of the tracheobronchial lymph nodes is not as easily accomplished without cross-sectional imaging because of superimposition of surrounding structures. Staging of primary lung tumors and determination of the tracheobronchial lymph node status are important for accurate prognostication [36–38]. CT was recently shown as a more accurate means (93%) of detecting tracheobronchial lymph node metastasis from primary lung tumors than radiography (57%) [36].

Metastatic lung disease. Similarly, CT is useful for detection of pulmonary metastasis. A recent retrospective study of 18 dogs found that only 9% of CT-detected pulmonary nodules were identified on thoracic radiographs and that nodules were detected in significantly more lung lobes using CT compared with radiographs [39]. The threshold for detection of pulmonary nodules is significantly lower with CT compared with survey radiography, although only 56% of pulmonary nodules less than 5 mm in diameter were identified by at least 1 of 10 radiologists in one study of metastatic canine osteosarcoma [40].

Mediastinal tumors. For masses within the mediastinum, CT can assist in discrimination between solid, fatty, cystic calcified, or vascular structures without superimposition of surrounding structures [41,42]. A recent study of CT features of canine and feline mediastinal masses found this procedure helpful for staging purposes, but it demonstrated no clinically exploitable relation between CT appearance and histology [42]. Further, the invasiveness of mediastinal masses on CT does not always correlate with findings at surgery and may not always predict the ease or difficulty of surgical resection.

Intra-abdominal neoplasia. CT has also been explored for staging of neoplasia involving various intra-abdominal organs, such as spleen, adrenal, and kidney, and is particularly useful when tumors include or are partially obscured by aerated lung or bone [12]. Staging of pheochromocytomas and adrenocortical tumors using CT has been described as useful in evaluating local invasion of surrounding vasculature and determining candidacy for surgical removal [43–45]. A study using CT to evaluate canine splenic masses found that malignant tumors had significantly lower HU values compared with nonmalignant masses with and without contrast medium administration, which is useful for preoperative prognostication and surgical planning [46]. Several descriptive studies also report on CT findings in dogs and cats with renal tumors [47–49].

Neoplasia of the integument and extremities. CT is helpful for clinical staging of tumors involving the skin or extremities, especially if radiotherapy or surgery is planned. CT more accurately defined tumor invasiveness and size than survey radiography or ultrasonography in one study of subcutaneous neoplasms with varying histologic findings [50]. Similarly, CT was successfully used to stage infiltrative lipoma in 22 dogs before surgery to determine an appropriate surgical approach or plan for definitive radiation therapy [51].

For feline vaccine site sarcomas, CT is the current staging method of choice to plan appropriate therapeutic intervention. The volume of tumor defined by CT far exceeded the grossly palpable volume of disease in one study [52]. Based on the soft tissue invasiveness of these tumors, it would seem that MRI might be a better choice compared with CT; however, these comparisons have yet to be made.

MRI

Technical advances

Although not as common as CT, MRI is becoming an important modality for veterinary medicine. Today, most veterinary teaching hospitals and many private specialty practices have access to MRI. The principles of image formation with MRI are not based on the attenuation of an x-ray beam as in CT but are based on the chemical and physical states of the tissue. MRI has the highest contrast resolution of all diagnostic imaging modalities. MRI scans can be acquired in any desired plane without changing the patient's position or without the need for multiplane reconstruction, thus avoiding loss of image quality.

MRI is superior to CT in its ability to distinguish difference in soft tissues, making it an excellent modality to evaluate tumors arising within soft tissue structures. Over the past several years, image sequences have been improved to aid in lesion detection and characterization. In addition to the three traditional spin echo pulse sequences (T1 weighted, T2 weighted, and proton density weighted), there are many other sequences that are commonly used to define the neoplastic lesion. Short time inversion recovery (STIR) sequences can be used to identify neoplastic lesions adjacent to fat. The typically hyperintense neoplastic lesion is made more conspicuous by suppressing the signal intensity from the surrounding fat. Fluid attenuation inversion recovery (FLAIR) is another sequence that is useful when the lesion in question is difficult to define because of the presence of adjacent or surrounding fluid. This sequence suppresses the signal from the fluid but not from the lesion.

The major limitation of MRI is still the initial cost of the equipment and the annual maintenance cost. There are two major types of MRI scanners: those with permanent magnets and those with superconductive magnets. MRI scanners with superconductive magnets have more capabilities as far as image sequences and have superior image quality, but their initial and annual maintenance costs are considerably higher. The MRI scanners with permanent magnets are not as expensive to purchase and have lower annual maintenance costs. They may also have an open gantry design, which makes it easier to access the patient during study, but they tend to have poorer image quality, especially when imaging small patients or small body parts. Currently, the choice between CT and MRI in veterinary medicine is largely based on economics and availability.

Clinical applications

Brain and spinal/paraspinal tumors. MRI is currently the preferred modality for detection, staging, and management of malignancy within the CNS. Several recent studies of MRI of CNS neoplasia demonstrate the utility of this modality for diagnosis and correlate MRI findings with histopathologic diagnoses [53–59]. Characteristic features, such as growth pattern, presence of edema, contrast enhancement, signal intensity pattern, and anatomic site, were identified to facilitate diagnosis and prognosis of intracranial tumors [59]. Because of overlapping features of different histologic subtypes, however, accurate prediction of tumor type based on MRI features is not always possible. Several MRI signs can be used to distinguish between neoplastic and nonneoplastic diseases, such as lesion shape, dural contact, dural tail sign, contrast enhancement, and invasion of adjacent bone [55]. For tumors of the spine and spinal cord, MRI was also useful in lesion localization and assessment of bone infiltration. In one study, sagittal T2-weighted images were most useful in anatomic localization, whereas transverse T1-weighted images with and without contrast administration were most helpful for localization and determination of tumor invasiveness [60].

Non-central nervous system tumors of the head and neck. Although most veterinary MRI literature pertains to neuroimaging, this modality is being used increasingly for the diagnosis or staging of head and neck tumors. The ability to obtain multiplanar cross-sectional images while avoiding superimposition of bony structures, coupled with superior soft tissue contrast, makes MRI an attractive modality in this setting.

MRI provided more accurate information regarding tumor size and invasion of adjacent structures but was similar to CT in delineation of bony involvement for a series of dogs with intraoral tumors [61]. CT was shown to be superior in this study for specific changes within bone, such as calcification and cortical erosion. MRI was superior to nasal radiography for evaluating tumor size and providing accurate staging information because of superior soft tissue contrast, but no large-scale study comparing MRI and CT for intranasal tumors has been published [62]. One report of MRI of multilobular tumor of bone of the skull in three dogs found this technique helpful in determination of the extent of brain and soft tissue involvement when planning surgical resection [63]. The same could be stated for tumors of the orbit, retrobulbar space, and ear. Availability and cost still make CT a more common choice for cross-sectional imaging of non-CNS head and neck tumors.

Abdominal neoplasia. Few studies describe the accuracy of MRI in assessment of suspected or known intra-abdominal neoplasia. One study of 35 focal splenic or hepatic lesions found MRI to be 94% accurate in differentiating benign from malignant splenic lesions, with a sensitivity and specificity of 100% and 90%, respectively [64]. As availability of MRI equipment increases, the use of MRI in staging, planning of biopsy procedures or surgical intervention, and monitoring response to therapy is likely to increase.

Neoplasia of the integument and extremities. MRI is commonly used in human patients for imaging of extremities, mainly for orthopedic indications and assessment of ligamentous and soft tissue injuries because of its superior soft tissue contrast. In veterinary patients, increasing availability and expertise in MRI should support the routine use of this modality in imaging neoplasia of the musculoskeletal system. A comparison study of amputated limbs from dogs with osteosarcoma found that CT was most accurate at predicting tumor length when intramedullary fibrosis was taken into account but did underestimate tumor length in one case. MRI measurements were less accurate but did not underestimate tumor length in any limb. This is important, because underestimation of tumor length can lead directly to treatment failure in limb-sparing procedures for osteosarcoma [65]. Another study of appendicular osteosarcoma found MRI more accurate when compared with scintigraphy or CT and reported that MRI had less of a tendency to overestimate tumor length than other imaging modalities [66]. MRI is the modality of choice in planning limb salvage procedures in human patients, and these data support this conclusion in dogs as well [65].

POSITRON EMISSION TOMOGRAPHY AND POSITRON EMISSION TOMOGRAPHY/CT

Technical Aspects of Positron Emission Tomography and Positron Emission Tomography/CT

PET technology was first used in the 1980s for diseases of the brain and heart through the mapping of glucose metabolism [67]. PET is now widely used for the staging and management of patients who have cancer, based on increased glucose transport and metabolism in tumors compared with surrounding normal tissues [67,68]. PET technology uses positron-emitting radionuclides tagged to biologically important molecules known to be involved in disease pathophysiology as markers or participants. Thus, PET is a functional imaging modality that is useful in characterizing physiologic processes, such as blood flow or glucose metabolism; visualizing ongoing biochemical and metabolic activities of normal or abnormal tissues; and assisting in drug development [69]. In oncology, the main focus is currently on detection and staging of malignancy, but the extent to which this technology could be useful in assessing response to therapy is also being explored.

Physics of positron emission tomography and positron-emitting radiopharmaceutic agents

The images produced by PET use the unique physical properties of positron-emitting radionuclides [70]. Multiple steps are involved in obtaining images with PET, beginning with the selection and production of an appropriate molecular probe through the labeling of a pharmaceutic agent or substrate with a positron-emitting radionuclide [71]. The positron emitted from the nucleus loses energy through collision with electrons in the surrounding tissue until it annihilates with an electron, producing two photons that are emitted approximately 180° apart [70,71]. The PET camera, designed to detect the pair of annihilation photons from the decay of the positron-emitting isotope, is composed of a ring of block detectors. The annihilation photons are captured in coincidence by opposing detectors that record "true" coincidence events, wherein a true coincidence is defined by a pair of unscattered photons arising from a single annihilation [71]. These paired events are stored in matrices or sinograms. An image reconstruction algorithm is applied to the sinograms to recover the radioactivity distribution, thus indirectly mapping the functional process created by the distribution of the radionuclide. The resulting images represent radiopharmaceutic accumulation in specific areas of the body closely related to the underlying biologic process of interest (Fig. 1). In the case of 2-deoxy-2-[^{18}F]fluoro-D-glucose (FDG), this would indicate areas of active glucose metabolism. Other radionuclides are used in PET, such as ^{11}C, ^{13}N, and ^{15}O, but because of their shorter half-lives, their use in clinical patients is limited. ^{18}F-labeled biomarkers, with a half-life of 110 minutes, can be transported from the cyclotron to the patient within a clinically reasonable time frame [67].

Labeling of substances with positron emitters allows specific biologic processes, such as glucose metabolism or DNA synthesis, to be mapped within tissues. The most common radiopharmaceutic agent used in modern PET imaging is FDG. Developed in 1976 for the purpose of mapping regional cerebral glucose metabolism, this molecule is an analogue of glucose that is used to quantify the rate at which the hexokinase reaction of glycolysis is occurring in a tissue or organ [72]. The development of this compound is based on the intracellular fate of 2-deoxyglucose (2-DG), an analogue of glucose that is phosphorylated in a similar manner by the hexokinase enzyme, the first step of glycolysis. Once phosphorylated, however, 2-DG-6-P is not a substrate for glucose phosphate isomerase; it is therefore trapped within the cell, unable to undergo the ensuing steps of glycolysis or the pentose phosphate shunt.

FDG is synthesized by replacing the hydrogen molecule at the C-2 position of 2-DG with ^{18}F. Phosphorylated FDG, just as 2-DG-6-P, cannot be further

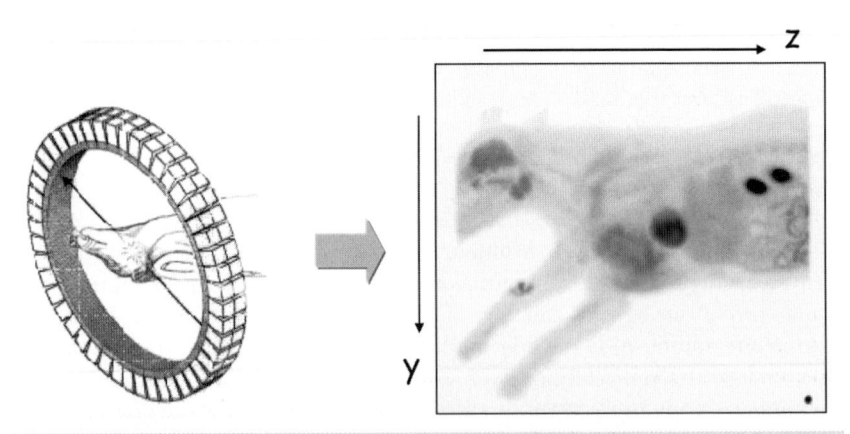

Fig. 1. After injection of the labeled radiopharmaceutic agent and the detection of a pair of annihilation photons in coincidence by a multiring PET camera, the events are collected and placed in sinograms. After reconstruction, a whole-body image is produced, mapping the uptake of the radionuclide throughout the patient. This image depicts a dog in right lateral recumbency with a large mast cell tumor involving the left axilla, within which significant uptake of radionuclide is visible. The site of 2-deoxy-2-[^{18}F]fluoro-D-glucose (FDG) is visible on the right antebrachium. (*Courtesy of* Bjoern Jakoby, MS, Knoxville, TN.)

metabolized; thus, all accumulated radioactivity over time is proportional to the rate of the hexokinase reaction in the observed tissue. At steady-state conditions in the absence of significant glucose-6 phosphatase activity, which dephosphorylates glucose and FDG, this represents the rate of glycolysis in the tissue [72].

Historically, a drawback of PET has been poor spatial resolution (ie, ability to resolve structures smaller than 1 cm in diameter). The intrinsic spatial resolution of a PET scanner is limited by the physics of positron emission and the detector design. This has significantly improved over the early single-slice scanners, which had a spatial resolution of greater than 15 mm. Currently, large-bore multislice PET scanners have a resolution of around 4 to 5 mm. Smaller laboratory animal–designed scanners are available with a spatial resolution of 1 to 2 mm and, more recently, with submillimeter resolution [67,73]. The fusion of PET with CT has ameliorated many of these issues, because the combination of these two modalities provides the best of both worlds: functional data coupled with high-resolution anatomic data.

Positron emission tomography/CT fusion

Great interest in fusing PET and CT images for lesion localization was born out of the relatively poor spatial resolution of PET and the excellent anatomic detail obtained with CT. This can be accomplished through visual, software-based, or hardware-based methods. Visual image fusion is simply viewing both studies side by side, whereas software-based image fusion requires computer programming to coregister the two data sets. This approach can work well for regions, such as the brain, where the skull provides fixed bony landmarks for fusion without appreciable organ movement during data acquisition. Recent hardware-based fusion of PET with CT has been an important step in maximizing the attributes of both modalities [70,73]. Since the first proof-of-concept combined scanner became operational in 1998, PET/CT has become the fastest growing imaging modality worldwide, with 500 to 1000 new systems installed in 2004 alone [74]. The fused scanner design allows anatomy and function to be assessed in a single scan session with single positioning of the patient, minimization of organ movement, and no requirement for labor-intensive image registration algorithms as when the scans are obtained separately [70]. Anatomic localization of functional abnormalities is difficult with PET alone; therefore, accurately aligned fused images of anatomy and function obtained with PET/CT offer substantial advantage to the study interpreter through the accurate localization of tracer accumulation, the distinction of normal uptake from pathologic examination, and the verification that a suspicious finding on one modality can be confirmed by the other modality [70].

Another advantage of PET/CT is the ability to use the CT data to correct the PET images for photon attenuation by tissues and organs. With conventional PET scanners, attenuation correction is accomplished by obtaining a "transmission scan" by rotating a radioactive source, typically ^{68}Ge, around the patient. With PET/CT fusion, the time for this additional scan is omitted, thus decreasing the total scan time by 25% to 30%. This results in more efficient use of fast-decaying PET radiopharmaceuticals [74].

Practical aspects of positron emission tomography and positron emission tomography/CT imaging

In human oncology, routine patient preparation involves fasting for approximately 6 hours before FDG injection to maximize uptake of the tracer by the tumor. After injection, it is important that the patient remains still and quiet for 60 to 90 minutes while FDG uptake occurs so as to avoid active skeletal muscle uptake of FDG as an interpretive pitfall [75]. FDG is injected into a peripheral vein, because use of a central line has been associated with retained activity in the line itself, leading to reconstruction streak artifacts. In the authors' experience with veterinary patients, fasting and use of a sedative premedicant with cage confinement are recommended after FDG injection to minimize aberrant uptake of FDG in skeletal muscle. Generally, PET scans, similar to CT or MRI, are performed under general anesthesia in veterinary patients. The impact of general anesthesia on FDG uptake and distribution is unknown if FDG is injected after anesthetic induction.

The use of intravenous or oral CT contrast agents in PET/CT is controversial because of concern about erroneous attenuation values in the correction of the PET images. In clinical practice, however, there is no demonstrable negative impact on image interpretation with oral or intravenous contrast use [76]. In the case of a potential artifact, which is most commonly noted within blood vessels, the non–attenuation-corrected images can be used to rule out a focus of increased tracer uptake as a neoplastic lesion (David Townsend, PhD, personal communication, 2007).

Image interpretation in positron emission tomography and positron emission tomography/CT

Uptake of FDG as a marker of glucose metabolism can be semiquantified using the standardized uptake value (SUV), which is used to determine the relative significance of uptake. The SUV is obtained by quantifying the radioactivity within a region of interest (ROI) placed over the lesion, taking the ratio of the ROI value (in microCi/mL) to the injected dose, divided by the patient's body weight.

$$SUV = \frac{\mu Ci/mL \text{ within ROI}}{\text{total } \mu Ci \text{ injected/weight}}$$

Uptake of FDG is not specific to cancer, and normal organs, such as brain, liver, spleen, tonsils, thymus, salivary glands, urinary system, and bone marrow, are known to have varying degrees of FDG uptake [75]. There are ranges of SUV values that are typically observed in areas of postoperative scarring, inflammation, infection, or neoplasia. Generally, an SUV greater than 2 is considered suspicious for malignancy [77]. A tissue biopsy is still needed for definitive diagnosis, but a PET scan can be important in decision making for patients having untreated or recurrent cancers.

Clinical Applications

PET imaging using FDG has become a routine part of the diagnostic evaluation of certain human cancers. Tumor cells have increased uptake of glucose; therefore, even though FDG is nonspecific for cancer, it is used for whole-body assessment of patients having suspected or confirmed neoplasia [68,71]. Numerous studies demonstrate the accuracy and value of PET in staging known neoplastic disease [78–80]. PET is also uniquely suited to detect recurrent disease and distinguish it from posttreatment fibrosis, scar, or necrosis. This is especially important for those tumors that require invasive biopsy techniques, such as brain tumors, or for those with a high rate of local and distant metastasis, such as breast or colorectal carcinomas [67].

Lack of available equipment and high cost of PET radiopharmaceutic agents have limited the use of PET as a diagnostic tool in veterinary oncology. Reports of PET and PET/CT in animals are sparse in the veterinary literature [81–83]. Feasibility reports of 2-DG and [^{3}H]-thymidine uptake in rodent tumor models and spontaneous canine tumors first appeared in 1981 [81,82]. PET imaging using ^{18}F-labeled monoclonal Fab fragment in four dogs with

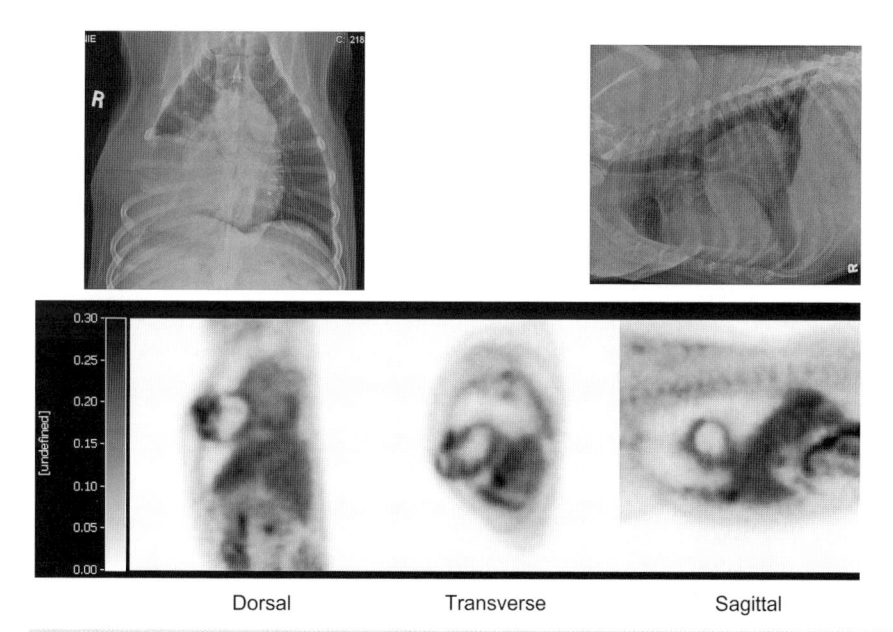

Fig. 2. Images obtained with conventional thoracic radiography (*top*) and whole-body FDG-PET (*bottom*; dorsal, transverse, and sagittal) from a dog with a large thoracic wall hemangiosarcoma. (*Courtesy of* Bjoern Jakoby, MS, Knoxville, TN.)

osteosarcoma was also reported [83]. PET was used to characterize experimentally induced and naturally occurring blastomycosis and was compared with cases of canine lymphoma, wherein lesions caused by blastomycosis were found to have higher SUVs than lesions caused by lymphoma in dogs with spontaneous disease [84,85]. Recently, PET studies using ^{18}F-fluoromisonidazole and ^{15}O-H$_2$0 were performed to evaluate tumor hypoxia and tumor perfusion, respectively, in canine soft tissue sarcoma [86]. PET was also used to image a dog with pulmonary carcinoma after treatment with intensity-modulated radiation therapy [87].

In our experience, many common canine tumors can be successfully imaged with PET. The authors have scanned cases of canine cutaneous mast cell tumor, multicentric and cutaneous lymphoma, mammary carcinoma, and hemangiosarcoma with a prototype large field-of-view scanner to determine the avidity of various tumors for FDG and assess the sensitivity and specificity of PET compared with anatomic imaging studies (radiography, CT, and ultrasound) for staging these malignancies. Fig. 2 illustrates an example of how FDG-PET was used in the staging of a dog with a large thoracic wall mass,

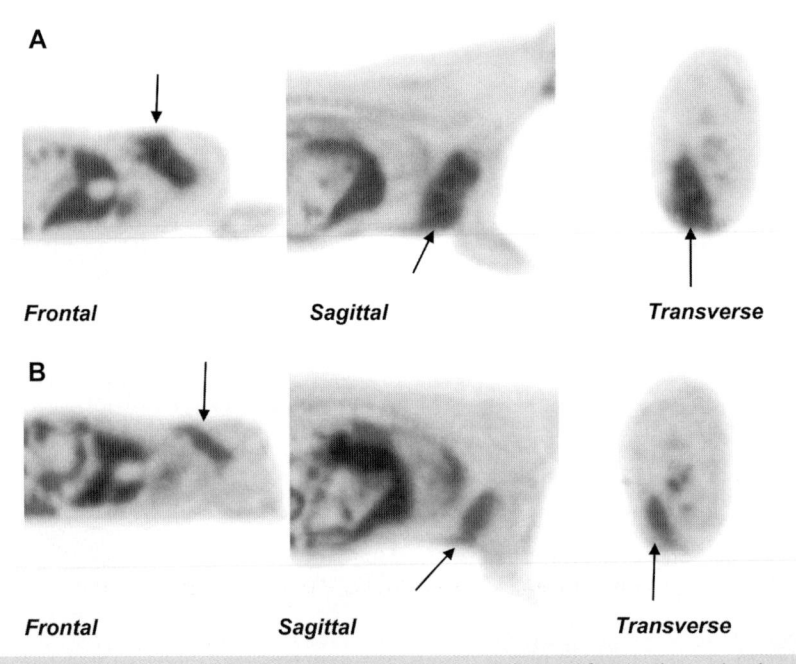

Fig. 3. FDG-PET images (frontal, sagittal, and transverse) obtained from a dog with a large grade II mast cell tumor in the right axillary region injected with FDG (2.55 mCi) using a 15-minute scan time and one bed position. (A) Images were created at the time of tumor staging, with thin arrows highlighting the tumor. (B) Images are after one dose of CCNU chemotherapy, demonstrating significant reduction in FDG uptake in the area of the tumor. (*Courtesy of* Bjoern Jakoby, MS, Knoxville, TN).

from which a biopsy confirmed hemangiosarcoma. Note the "cold" center of FDG uptake within the mass, representative of a blood-filled cavity within the tumor with minimal metabolic activity. Fig. 3 demonstrates how FDG-PET was used to detect response to CCNU chemotherapy in a dog with a non-resectable, grade II mast cell tumor of the right axilla. Note that the diffuse area of increased FDG uptake is significantly reduced 3 weeks after the initial dose of chemotherapy. Currently, the availability of PET or PET/CT for staging and evaluation of response to therapy in veterinary patients is limited to a few locations in the United States and Europe.

SUMMARY

The widespread use and collective experience with CT and MRI in veterinary medicine represent an important advance in the care for companion animals with cancer. PET is an important imaging modality that has changed the practice of human oncology in the past decade, improving the treatment of malignancy through enhancing the accuracy of staging and detection of residual disease. With greater availability, PET and PET/CT fusion are expected to join the ranks of CT and MRI in the near future for the benefit of tumor-bearing pets.

References

[1] Van Camp S, Fisher P, Thrall DE. Dynamic CT measurement of contrast medium wash-in kinetics in canine nasal tumors. Vet Radiol Ultrasound 2000;41(5):403–8.
[2] Pollard RE, Garcia TC, Stieger SM, et al. Quantitative evaluation of perfusion and permeability of peripheral tumors using contrast-enhanced computed tomography. Invest Radiol 2004;39(6):340–9.
[3] Tidwell AS, Johnson KL. Computed tomography-guided percutaneous biopsy: criteria for accurate needle tip identification. Vet Radiol Ultrasound 1994;35(6):440–4.
[4] Tidwell AS, Johnson KL. Computed tomography-guided percutaneous biopsy in the dog and cat: description of the technique and preliminary evaluation in 14 patients. Vet Radiol Ultrasound 1994;35(6):445–56.
[5] Vignoli M, Ohlerth S, Rossi F, et al. Computed tomography-guided fine-needle aspiration and tissue-core biopsy of bone lesions in small animals. Vet Radiol Ultrasound 2004;45(2):125–30.
[6] Fike JR, LeCouteur RA, Cann CE, et al. Computerized tomography of brain tumors of the rostral and middle fossas in the dog. Am J Vet Res 1981;42(2):275–81.
[7] Mandelker L. Using a computed brain and orbital tomography to diagnose a brain tumor in a dog. Vet Med Small Anim Clin 1981;76(8):1164–7.
[8] Swengel JR. Computerized tomography for diagnosis of brain tumor in a dog. J Am Vet Med Assoc 1982;181(6):605.
[9] Turrel JM, Fike JR, LeCouteur RA, et al. Computed tomographic characteristics of primary brain tumors in 50 dogs. J Am Vet Med Assoc 1986;188(8):851–6.
[10] LeCouteur RA. Current concepts in the diagnosis and treatment of brain tumors in dogs and cats. J Small Anim Pract 1999;40(9):411–6.
[11] Kraft SL, Gavin PR. Intracranial neoplasia. Clin Tech Small Anim Pract 1999;14(2):112–23.
[12] Wisner ER, Pollard RE. Trends in veterinary cancer imaging. Veterinary and Comparative Oncology 2004;2(2):49–74.
[13] Koblik PD, LeCouteur RA, Higgins RJ, et al. CT-guided brain biopsy using a modified Pelorus Mark III stereotactic system: experience with 50 dogs. Vet Radiol Ultrasound 1999;40(5):434–50.

[14] Koblik PD, LeCouteur RA, Higgins RJ, et al. Modification and application of a Pelorus Mark III stereotactic system for CT-guided brain biopsy in 50 dogs. Vet Radiol Ultrasound 1999;40(5):424–33.
[15] Moissonnier P, Blot S, Devauchelle P, et al. Stereotactic CT-guided brain biopsy in the dog. J Small Anim Pract 2002;43(3):115–23.
[16] Giroux A, Jones JC, Bohn JH, et al. A new device for stereotactic CT-guided biopsy of the canine brain: design, construction, and needle placement accuracy. Vet Radiol Ultrasound 2002;43(3):229–36.
[17] Forrest LJ, Mackie TR, Ruchala K, et al. The utility of megavoltage computed tomography images from a helical tomotherapy system for setup verification purposes. Int J Radiat Oncol Biol Phys 2004;60(5):1639–44.
[18] Rohrer Bley C, Blattman H, Roos M, et al. Assessment of a radiotherapy patient immobilization device using single plane port radiographs and a remote computed tomography scanner. Vet Radiol Ultrasound 2003;44(4):470–5.
[19] Lester NV, Hopkins AL, Bova FJ, et al. Radiosurgery using a stereotactic headframe system for irradiation of brain tumors in dogs. J Am Vet Med Assoc 2001;219(11): 1562–7.
[20] Rudich SR, Feeney DA, Anderson KL, et al. Computed tomography of masses of the brachial plexus and contributing nerve roots in dogs. Vet Radiol Ultrasound 2004;45(1): 46–50.
[21] Essman SC, Hoover JP, Bahr RJ, et al. An intrathoracic malignant peripheral nerve sheath tumor in a dog. Vet Radiol Ultrasound 2002;43(3):255–9.
[22] Niles JD, Dyce J, Mattoon JS. Computed tomography for the diagnosis of lumbosacral nerve sheath tumor and management by hemipelvectomy. J Small Anim Pract 2001;42(5): 248–52.
[23] Pease AP, Berry CR, Mott JP, et al. Radiographic, computed tomographic and histopathologic appearance of a presumed spinal cord chordoma in a dog. Vet Radiol Ultrasound 2002;43(4):338–42.
[24] Park RD, Beck ER, LeCouteur RA. Comparison of computed tomography and radiography for detecting changes induced by malignant nasal neoplasia in dogs. J Am Vet Med Assoc 1992;201(11):1720–4.
[25] Lefebvre J, Kuehn NF, Wortinger A. Computed tomography as an aid in the diagnosis of chronic nasal disease in dogs. J Small Anim Pract 2005;46(6):280–5.
[26] Rassnick KM, Goldkamp CE, Erb HN, et al. Evaluation of factors associated with survival in dogs with untreated nasal carcinomas: 139 cases (1993–2003). J Am Vet Med Assoc 2006;229(3):401–6.
[27] Codner EC, Lurus AG, Miller JB, et al. Comparison of computed tomography with radiography as a noninvasive diagnostic technique for chronic nasal disease in dogs. J Am Vet Med Assoc 1993;202(7):1106–10.
[28] Kuehn NF. Nasal computed tomography. Clin Tech Small Anim Pract 2006;21(2): 55–9.
[29] Schoenborn WC, Wisner ER, Kass PP, et al. Retrospective assessment of computed tomographic imaging of feline sinonasal disease in 62 cats. Vet Radiol Ultrasound 2003;44(2):185–95.
[30] Tromblee TC, Jones JC, Etue AE, et al. Association between clinical characteristics, computed tomography characteristics, and histologic diagnosis for cats with sinonasal disease. Vet Radiol Ultrasound 2006;47(3):241–8.
[31] Liptak JM, Withrow SJ. Withrow and MacEwen's small animal clinical oncology. In: Withrow SJ, Vail DM, editors. Surgical approach to oral tumors use of CT 4th edition. St. Louis (MO): Saunders/Elsevier; 2007.
[32] Hathcock JT, Newton JC. Computed tomographic characteristics of multilobular tumor of bone involving the cranium in 7 dogs and zygomatic arch in 2 dogs. Vet Radiol Ultrasound 2000;41(3):214–7.

[33] Lascelles BD, Thomson MJ, Dernell WS, et al. Combined dorsolateral and intraoral approach for the resection of tumors of the maxilla in the dog. J Am Anim Hosp Assoc 2003;39(3):294–305.

[34] Mouatt JG, Straw RC. Use of mandibular symphysiotomy to allow extensive caudal hemimaxillectomy in a dog. Aust Vet J 2002;80(5):272–6.

[35] Mouatt JG. Acrylic cranioplasty and axial pattern flap following calvarial and cerebral mass excision in a dog. Aust Vet J 2002;80(4):211–5.

[36] Paoloni MC, Adams WM, Dubielzig RR, et al. Comparison of computed tomography and radiography with histopathologic findings in tracheobronchial lymph nodes in dogs with primary lung tumors: 14 cases (1999–2002). J Am Vet Med Assoc 2006;228(11): 1718–22.

[37] Ogilvie GK, Weigel RM, Haschek WM, et al. Prognostic factors for tumor remission and survival in dogs after surgery for primary lung tumor: 76 cases (1975–1985). J Am Vet Med Assoc 1989;195(1):109–12.

[38] McNiel EA, Ogilvie GK, Powers BE, et al. Evaluation of prognostic factors for dogs with primary lung tumors: 67 cases (1985–1992). J Am Vet Med Assoc 1997;211(11): 1422–7.

[39] Nemanic S, London CA, Wisner ER. Comparison of thoracic radiographs and single breath-hold helical CT for detection of pulmonary nodules in dogs with metastatic neoplasia. J Vet Intern Med 2006;20(3):508–15.

[40] Waters DJ, Coakley FV, Cohen MD, et al. The detection of pulmonary metastases by helical CT: a clinicopathologic study in dogs. J Comput Assist Tomogr 1998;22(2): 235–40.

[41] Prather AB, Berry CR, Thrall DE. Use of radiography in combination with computed tomography for the assessment of noncardiac thoracic disease in the dog and cat. Vet Radiol Ultrasound 2005;46(2):114–21.

[42] Yoon J, Feeney DA, Cronk DE, et al. Computed tomographic evaluation of canine and feline mediastinal masses in 14 patients. Vet Radiol Ultrasound 2004;45(6):542–6.

[43] Hylands R. Veterinary diagnostic imaging: malignant pheochromocytoma of the left adrenal gland invading the caudal vena cava, accompanied by a cortisol secreting adrenocortical carcinoma of the right adrenal gland. Can Vet J 2005;46(12):1156–8.

[44] Rosenstein DS. Diagnostic imaging in canine pheochromocytoma. Vet Radiol Ultrasound 2000;41(6):499–506.

[45] Voorhout G, Stolp R, Rijnberk A, et al. Assessment of survey radiography and comparison with x-ray computed tomography for detection of hyperfunctioning adrenocortical tumors in dogs. J Am Vet Med Assoc 1990;196(11):1799–803.

[46] Fife WD, Samii VF, Drost WT, et al. Comparison between malignant and nonmalignant splenic masses in dogs using contrast-enhanced computed tomography. Vet Radiol Ultrasound 2004;45(4):289–97.

[47] Saridomichelakis MN, Koutinas CK, Souftas V, et al. Extensive caudal vena cava thrombosis secondary to unilateral renal tubular cell carcinoma in a dog. J Small Anim Pract 2004;45(2):108–12.

[48] Yamazoe K, Ohashi F, Kadosawa T, et al. Computed tomography of renal masses in dogs and cats. J Vet Med Sci 1994;56(4):813–6.

[49] Moe L, Lium B. Computed tomography of hereditary multifocal renal cystadenocarcinomas in German Shepherd dogs. Vet Radiol Ultrasound 1997;38(5):335–43.

[50] Hahn KA, Lantz GC, Salisbury SK, et al. Comparison of survey radiography with ultrasonography and x-ray computed tomography for clinical staging of subcutaneous neoplasms in dogs. J Am Vet Med Assoc 1990;196(11):1795–8.

[51] McEntee MC, Thrall DE. Computed tomographic imaging of infiltrative lipoma in 22 dogs. Vet Radiol Ultrasound 2001;42(3):221–5.

[52] McEntee MC, Page RL. Feline vaccine-associated sarcomas. J Vet Intern Med 2001;15(1): 176–82.

[53] Snyder JM, Shofer FS, Van Winkle TJ, et al. Canine intracranial neoplasia: 173 cases (1986–2003). J Vet Intern Med 2006;20:669–75.
[54] Sage JE, Samii VF, Abramson CJ, et al. Comparison of conventional spin-echo and fast spin-echo magnetic resonance imaging in the canine brain. Vet Radiol Ultrasound 2006;47: 249–53.
[55] Cherubini GB, Mantis P, Martinez TA, et al. Utility of magnetic resonance imaging for distinguishing neoplastic from non-neoplastic brain lesions in dogs and cats. Vet Radiol Ultrasound 2005;46:384–7.
[56] McDonnell JJ, Tidwell AS, Faissler D, et al. Magnetic resonance imaging features of cervical spinal cord meningiomas. Vet Radiol Ultrasound 2005;46:368–74.
[57] Troxel MT, Vie CH, Massicote C, et al. Magnetic resonance imaging features of feline intracranial neoplasia: retrospective analysis of 46 cats. J Vet Intern Med 2004;18: 176–89.
[58] Lipsitz D, Higgin RJ, Kortz GD, et al. Glioblastoma multiforme: clinical findings, magnetic resonance imaging, and pathology in five dogs. Vet Pathol 2003;40(6):659–69.
[59] Kraft SL, Gavin PR, DeHaan C, et al. Retrospective review of 50 canine intracranial tumors evaluated by magnetic resonance imaging. J Vet Intern Med 1997;11(4):218–25.
[60] Kippenes H, Gavin PR, Bagley RS, et al. Magnetic resonance imaging features of tumors of the spine and spinal cord in dogs. Vet Radiol Ultrasound 1999;40(6):627–33.
[61] Kafka UC, Carstens A, Steenkamp G, et al. Diagnostic value of magnetic resonance imaging and computed tomography for oral masses in dogs. J S Afr Vet Assoc 2004;75:163–8.
[62] Petite AF, Dennis R. Comparison of radiography and magnetic resonance imaging for evaluating the extent of nasal neoplasia in dogs. J Small Anim Pract 2006;47:529–36.
[63] Lipsitz D, Levitski RE, Berry WL. Magnetic resonance imaging features of multilobular osteochondrosarcoma in 3 dogs. Vet Radiol Ultrasound 2001;42(1):14–9.
[64] Clifford CA, Pretorius ES, Weisse C, et al. Magnetic resonance imaging of focal splenic and hepatic lesions in the dog. J Vet Intern Med 2004;18:330–8.
[65] Davis GJ, Kapatkin AS, Craig LE, et al. Comparison of radiography, computed tomography, and magnetic resonance imaging for evaluation of appendicular osteosarcoma in dogs. J Am Vet Med Assoc 2002;220:1171–6.
[66] Wallack ST, Wisner ER, Werner JA, et al. Accuracy of magnetic resonance imaging for estimating intramedullary osteosarcoma extent in pre-operative planning of canine limb-salvage procedures. Vet Radiol Ultrasound 2002;43:432–41.
[67] Rohren EM, Turkington TG, Coleman RE. Clinical applications of PET in oncology. Radiology 2004;231(2):305–32.
[68] Warburg O. On the origin of cancer cells. Science 1956;123:306–14.
[69] Alavi A, Kung JW, Zhuang H. Implications of PET based molecular imaging on the current and future practice of medicine. Semin Nucl Med 2004;34(1):56–69.
[70] Zanzonico P. Positron emission tomography: a review of basic principles, scanner design and performance, and current systems. Semin Nucl Med 2004;34(2):87–111.
[71] Townsend DW. Physical principles and technology of clinical PET imaging. Ann Acad Med Singapore 2004;33:133–45.
[72] Fowler JS, Ido T. Initial and subsequent approach for the synthesis of ^{18}FDG. Semin Nucl Med 2002;32(1):6–12.
[73] Townsend DW. From 3-D positron emission tomography to 3-D positron emission tomography/computed tomography: what did we learn? Mol Imaging Biol 2004;6(5):275–90.
[74] Von Schulthess GK, Steinert HC, Hany TF. Integrated PET/CT: current applications and future directions. Radiology 2006;238(2):405–22.
[75] Cook GJR, Wegner EA, Fogelman I. Pitfalls and artifacts in ^{18}FDG PET and PET/CT oncologic imaging. Semin Nucl Med 2004;34(2):122–33.
[76] Sachelarie I, Kerr K, Ghesani M, et al. Integrated PET-CT: evidence-based review of oncology indications. Oncology (Williston Park) 2005;19(4):481–90.

[77] Kumar R, Nadig MR, Chauhan A. Positron emission tomography: clinical applications in oncology. Expert Rev Anticancer Ther 2005;5(6):1079–94.
[78] Hustinix R, Benard F, Alavi A. Whole-body FDG-PET imaging in the management of patients with cancer. Semin Nucl Med 2002;32:35–46.
[79] Dobert N, Menzel C, Berner U, et al. Positron emission tomography in patients with Hodgkin's disease: correlation to histologic subtypes. Cancer Biother Radiopharm 2003;18(4): 565–71.
[80] Peterson JJ, Kransdorf MJ, O'Connor MI. Diagnosis of occult bone metastases: positron emission tomography. Clin Orthop 2003;415(Suppl):S120–8.
[81] Larson SM, Weiden PL, Grunbaum Z, et al. Positron imaging feasibility studies. I: characterization of [^{3}H]-thymidine uptake in rodent and canine neoplasms: concise communication. J Nucl Med 1981;22:869–74.
[82] Larson SM, Weiden PL, Grunbaum Z, et al. Positron imaging feasibility studies. II: characteristics of 2-deoxyglucose uptake in rodent and canine neoplasms: concise communication. J Nucl Med 1981;22:875–9.
[83] Page RL, Garg PK, Garg S, et al. PET imaging of osteosarcoma in dogs using a fluorine-18-labeled monoclonal antibody Fab fragment. J Nucl Med 1994;35:1506–13.
[84] Bassett CLM, Daniel GB, Legendre AM, et al. Characterization of uptake of 2-deoxy-2-[^{18}F]fluoro-D-glucose by fungal-associated inflammation: the standardized uptake value is greater for lesions of blastomycosis than for lymphoma in dogs with naturally occurring disease. Mol Imaging Biol 2002;4(3):201–7.
[85] Matwichuk CL, Daniel GB, Bowman LA, et al. Fluorine-18 fluorodeoxyglucose accumulation in Blastomyces dermatitidis-associated inflammation in a dog. Clin Positron Imaging 1999;2(4):217–21.
[86] Bruehlmeier M, Kaser-Hotz B, Achermann R, et al. Measurement of tumor hypoxia in spontaneous canine sarcomas. Vet Radiol Ultrasound 2005;46(4):348–54.
[87] Ballegeer EA, Forrest LJ, Jeraj R, et al. PET/CT following intensity-modulated radiation therapy for primary lung tumor in a dog. Vet Radiol Ultrasound 2006;47(2):228–33.

Chemotherapy: New Uses for Old Drugs

Anthony J. Mutsaers, DVM

Division of Molecular and Cell Biology, Sunnybrook Health Sciences Centre,
Department of Medical Biophysics, University of Toronto, S-221, 2075 Bayview Avenue,
Toronto, Ontario, M4N 3M5, Canada

The range of chemotherapeutic drug options available to veterinarians continues to expand as we learn how to translate them from human oncology to the treatment of our patients. Newer drugs, such as gemcitabine [1], ifosfamide [2], and vinorelbine [3], are just a few examples. In addition to this are different approaches that evaluate alternate ways to use chemotherapeutics. Examples include intracavitary applications that aid in malignant effusion control by pleurodesis [4] or radiation therapy sensitization [5], in which the benefits of the drugs are not necessarily restricted to their individual cancer cell cytotoxicity per se. Another approach that is emerging in the era of targeted cancer treatment is termed *metronomic* chemotherapy. This terminology was coined by Dr. Doug Hanahan and his colleagues in an editorial [6] regarding the publication of two preclinical studies in rodent models [7,8] in which there was a treatment advantage for chemotherapeutics delivered in a low-dose continuous manner, even in tumors previously made resistant to the same drug given in a more traditional schedule [6]. Other popular names for this approach include low-dose continuous chemotherapy or antiangiogenic chemotherapy. Regardless of the chosen terminology, this form of treatment is receiving increased attention in human and veterinary oncology circles. The use of drugs that we are already familiar with, plus the low cost, ease of application, and generally nontoxic nature of the dose and schedules chosen, make this approach attractive for application to veterinary oncology practice. The aim of this article is to outline the origin of and rationale for metronomic chemotherapy, explain what is known about the mechanism(s) responsible for its potential benefit, and highlight some of the clinical trial evaluations taking place. Although most metronomic clinical trials are taking place in human beings, veterinary oncology trials are also ongoing; thus, contacting a veterinary oncologist regarding the results of these trials, cases that may benefit, and specific protocols is advised.

E-mail address: anthony.mutsaers@sri.utoronto.ca

CHEMOTHERAPEUTIC DOSING: "HIGH TIME" FOR SOMETHING NEW?

To understand how metronomic chemotherapy is a departure from current strategies requires a brief review of the evolution of chemotherapeutic dosing. Most chemotherapy administration, especially for solid tumors, is based on the concept of giving the "maximum tolerated dose" (MTD). The rationale for this is based, in large part, on work by Skipper and colleagues [9] in the early 1970s, which demonstrated a logarithmic cancer cell kill with increasing drug concentration. Therefore, in theory, the more drug administered, the higher is the chance of total tumor eradication, and hence potential for cure. The limiting factor for the dose administered is the toxicity to normal noncancerous tissues, however, with the most commonly affected being rapidly dividing cells located in the bone marrow and intestinal tract. The result of this merging of the theoretic and practical has been an approach that seeks to deliver as much drug as can be tolerated by the patient (the MTD), followed by an inevitable break period to allow repair of damage to normal tissues. Over the years, the MTD strategy has intensified with improvements in supportive care agents, such as gastrointestinal protectants, antinausea medications, hematopoietic growth factors, and bone marrow transplantation. The result of the application of MTD chemotherapy, especially combination chemotherapy (which combines multiple drugs with differing mechanisms of action and nonoverlapping toxicity profiles), has been great extension of survival for several cancers and outright cure for some. The gains made with this approach have not resulted in cures for most of the common solid tumors, however, despite the application of dose-dense and bone marrow transplantation strategies.

What is the reason for this plateau in success? Although many theories exist, the scheduling limitations of MTD are of particular relevance [9–11]. The original dose-response studies by Skipper and colleagues [9] were performed in vitro, using log-phase nonmutagenic cells grown in monolayer culture. Although such a laboratory-based methodology continues to be applied to chemosensitivity screening for new compounds, this artificial system cannot take into account the complex tumor microenvironment that exists in the body. Cancer cells growing in a patient do not behave in a similar manner to those in a Petri dish, nor do they exist in isolation. The survival and growth of tumors are influenced by contributions from many molecules and other cell types (eg, stromal support structures, inflammatory cells, blood and lymphatic vessels) and by alterations in tissue oxygenation and interstitial fluid pressure (Fig. 1). Direct targeting of the interactions between a tumor cell and its microenvironment has been a major focus of research as a method to improve on results obtained with more traditional cancer therapies, such as surgery, radiation, and cytotoxic chemotherapy. The concept of metronomic chemotherapy has grown out of consideration of whether chemotherapeutics can alter the tumor microenvironment, in addition to the effects they have on the cancer cells themselves. It is hoped that by understanding the nature of chemotherapeutic effects on the tumor microenvironment, it may be possible to improve

Increased interstitial fluid pressure

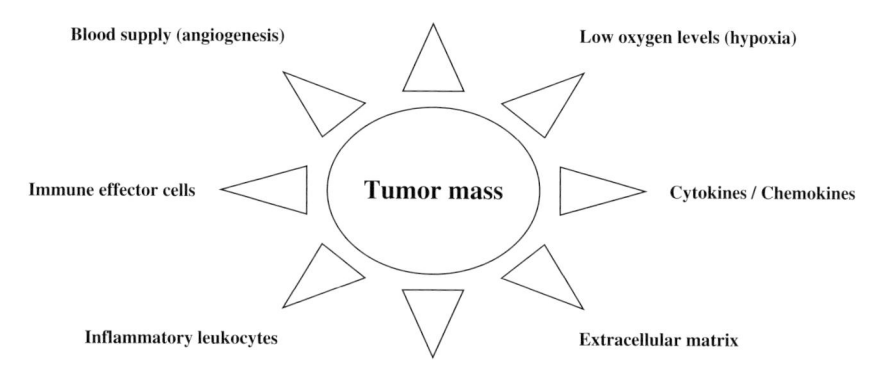

Blood supply (angiogenesis)　　　　　**Low oxygen levels (hypoxia)**

Immune effector cells　　　Tumor mass　　　**Cytokines / Chemokines**

Inflammatory leukocytes　　　　　**Extracellular matrix**

Stromal cells (e.g. fibroblasts)

Fig. 1. Tumor cells in vivo are influenced by numerous microenvironmental factors. Altering these components may potentiate tumor cell kill obtained using conventional chemotherapy approaches. Metronomic scheduling of chemotherapy inhibits angiogenesis, the tumor's growing blood supply.

on the overall antitumor effects of these drugs. As reviewed in this article, these effects seem to be related, at least in part, to suppression of the blood supply that develops to provide oxygen and nutrients and to remove waste products from growing tumors, a process known as tumor angiogenesis [12].

PHARMACOLOGY OF "METRONOMIC" CHEMOTHERAPY

The pharmacokinetics of chemotherapeutic dosing are often represented by a graph of drug concentration per unit time, with the desired expression of dose received represented by the area under the curve (AUC). Although the MTD approach seeks to push the dose administered as high as is possible, the metronomic approach can be thought of as delivering no more than the minimum amount required as frequently as possible and over a longer period (Fig. 2). Numerically, this concept could be illustrated in an extreme example as the possibility that giving the median effective concentration of drug (EC_{50}) for 30 days may be more effective than administering an amount that is 30-fold higher (eg, EC_{1500}) for 1 day in a monthly schedule, even though the calculated drug exposure would be equivalent for the two strategies [10].

The use of MTD chemotherapy involves a break period to allow for recovery of normal tissues from toxic side effects. The goal of metronomically delivered chemotherapy is elimination of the long break periods between doses, because it is during this time that exploitable alterations in tumor cells and their microenvironment occur. These changes include the tumor cell repopulation, hypoxia, and damage repair that are so familiar to radiation biologists and are key reasons for the delivery of radiation therapy in low, frequent, "metronomic" dosing schedules. Although this nickname is a relatively new one, the

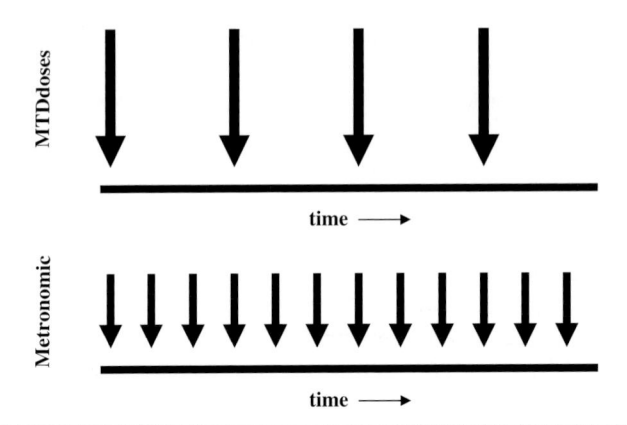

Fig. 2. The conceptual difference between MTD chemotherapy (*top*) and metronomic chemotherapy (*bottom*). Arrows represent each dose of chemotherapy administered, with the size of the arrow indicative of the amount of drug given. MTD-based chemotherapy involves a mandatory break period to allow for recovery from toxicity to normal tissues, whereas metronomic chemotherapy seeks to eliminate the break period with smaller and more frequent dosing.

concept itself is not necessarily so, because the reduced-dose, long-term, maintenance chemotherapy regimens that are an important part of standard therapies for certain cancers, such as childhood acute lymphoblastic leukemia, could also be considered a form of metronomic chemotherapy [10]. The reduction of the break period used in metronomic chemotherapy is also conceptually similar to the same practice used in hyperfractionated radiation therapy or newer dose-dense chemotherapy regimens. The important exception is that the goal is not necessarily to deliver a larger total amount of chemotherapy per unit time, as is the case with dose-dense chemotherapy. Rather, the focus remains on elimination of the break period [12].

METRONOMIC CHEMOTHERAPY AS AN ANTIANGIOGENIC STRATEGY

The aspect of tumor biology and microenvironment that has been studied most extensively with regard to metronomic chemotherapy is the process of tumor angiogenesis, defined earlier as the development and growth of a tumor's own blood supply. There certainly may be several mechanisms that play a contributing role; however, the antiangiogenic aspects of this therapy are thought to result from three major factors: (1) chemotherapy affects endothelial cells in a much more direct and selective manner compared with other cell and tissue types; (2) endothelial progenitor cells derived from the bone marrow seem to be directly targeted by metronomic chemotherapeutic scheduling; and (3) metronomic chemotherapy modulates the levels of angiogenic growth factors and inhibitors in favor of the latter, and therefore indirectly influences angiogenic balance [12]. Upregulation of the inhibitor thrombospondin-1 (TSP-1) seems to be a key molecule involved in this process; however, downregulation of important stimulatory factors, such as vascular endothelial growth factor (VEGF), may also be involved.

Selective Endothelial Cell Cytotoxicity

The effects of chemotherapy can be considered to be relatively nonselective in that the damage caused is most often preferentially inflicted on rapidly dividing cell populations. As a result, it is perhaps not surprising to find that many traditional chemotherapeutics act as antiangiogenic drugs simply because the endothelial cells that make up a tumor's growing blood supply are also highly proliferative, whereas most normal vasculature in the adult remains relatively quiescent [13]. Because clinical application of metronomic chemotherapy has been shown to be generally well tolerated by tissues normally sensitive to traditional MTD doses [13,14], the question arises as to why these rapidly dividing normal cell populations, such as bone marrow precursors and intestinal epithelial cells, are not similarly affected during metronomic treatments. In vitro laboratory experiments designed to compare the cytotoxicity of chemotherapy drugs against a variety of cell types clearly demonstrate inhibition of proliferation and migration of endothelial cells at picomolar drug concentrations [15–17]. The concentration of drugs, such as cyclophosphamide, methotrexate, vinblastine, and paclitaxel, that are required to produce similar effects in nonendothelial cell lines cells, such as tumor cells, epithelial cells, lymphocytes, and fibroblasts, are 10- to 100,000-fold higher, however. These effects demonstrate an apparent intrinsic sensitivity of endothelial cells to ultralow doses of chemotherapy and help to explain why normal tissues, even those with high numbers of proliferating cells, may be relatively spared during metronomic chemotherapy protocols, whereas new tumor blood vessels are selectively inhibited. The differential effects observed in the laboratory seem to be most pronounced with the microtubule inhibitors.

Circulating Endothelial Progenitor Cells

Until recently, it was thought that new endothelial cells were derived from local division of differentiated endothelial cells in preexisting vessels. Currently, the biology, proportion, and contribution of bone marrow-derived circulating endothelial progenitor cells to the process of tumor angiogenesis are the subject of much investigation and debate. These cells can be mobilized from the bone marrow, enter the peripheral circulation, home to sites of ongoing angiogenesis, incorporate into a lumen of a growing sprout, and differentiate into endothelial cells [18]. Because these cells are also mobilized out of the bone marrow in response to several proangiogenic molecules (eg, VEGF), they are also considered a target of antiangiogenic treatment strategies aimed at neutralizing these growth factors. These cells also seem to be direct targets of chemotherapy independent of whether the drugs are used in an MTD or metronomic fashion, however [19]. Specifically, circulating endothelial progenitor cell (CEP) levels decrease markedly and abruptly when MTD chemotherapy is administered, only to rebound rapidly during the break period between doses (similar to the hematopoietic rebound of other bone marrow precursor cells that are similarly affected, such as those in the granulocytic and thrombocytic lineages). This compensatory rebound in CEPs, and their consequent contribution to angiogenesis, was negated by metronomic scheduling of cyclophosphamide in a human lymphoma model in laboratory mice, in which the drug was administered at low weekly doses or continuously through the drinking water [19,20]. Although there is still much to learn regarding bone marrow–derived CEPs, if they make a significant contribution to angiogenesis, the continuous suppression of these cells could represent a major component of the antiangiogenic mechanisms of metronomic chemotherapy.

Importantly, CEPs can be measured and quantified in the bloodstream. This tool has allowed them to be investigated as a noninvasive marker of angiogenesis [21–23]. A significant challenge to the application of metronomic chemotherapy is determination of the optimal dose, because the chosen dose is not guided by predictable toxicities, such as myelosuppression. Monitoring CEPs has decreased the empiricism associated with metronomic dosing [21]; this technique is now used in metronomic therapy clinical trials. Importantly, an assay of CEPs using flow cytometry has been developed for dogs and could potentially be incorporated as a biomarker into future veterinary trials of metronomic chemotherapy or other antiangiogenic strategies [24].

Growth/Survival Factor Modulation

Angiogenesis is a tightly regulated process involving a balance between numerous proangiogenic and antiangiogenic endogenous factors [25]. It is widely accepted that for a solid tumor to develop its own blood supply, the balance must be tipped in favor of angiogenic stimulation. This process, referred to as the "angiogenic switch," is often associated with mutational changes that occur with cancer progression [26]. Because of this balance, antiangiogenic treatment strategies often directly target these stimulators or inhibitors by attempting to suppress the former or boost the latter. As an example, the first US Food and Drug Administration (FDA)–approved targeted antiangiogenic drug in oncology, bevacizumab (Avastin), is an antibody against human VEGF, which is considered to be one of the most potent angiogenic growth factors [12,25].

Two independent studies have demonstrated that elevation of the endogenous angiogenesis inhibitor TSP-1 may be one factor associated with metronomic chemotherapy dosing [27,28]. This molecule interacts with a receptor on endothelial cells (CD36) that is not found on other cell types, such as hematopoietic stem cells. Upregulation of TSP-1 was demonstrated in cultured endothelial cells exposed to low doses of 4-hydroxy-cyclophosphamide, and the anticancer effect of metronomic therapy with cyclophosphamide was lost when experiments were conducted in TSP-1 knockout (Tsp1-null) mice. Further, a synergistic effect has been observed when metronomic chemotherapy was combined with ABT510, a peptide derivative of TSP-1, in the PC-3 prostatic carcinoma model in mice [29]. These results suggest that metronomic chemotherapy, independent of whether or not it upregulates TSP-1 itself, may complement the antiangiogenic effects of this inhibitor molecule. The results of a recent human clinical trial using metronomic cyclophosphamide and etoposide in pediatric cancer patients showed that elevated TSP-1 levels correlated with prolonged response [30]. It is not known if these levels were induced by therapy or if patients had increased endogenous levels irrespective of treatment. In either case, a possible implication supported by preclinical studies is that metronomic chemotherapy potentiates the beneficial effects of TSP-1 [31]. Treatment with the TSP-1–derived peptide ABT510 or ABT526 is currently undergoing phase II clinical trial evaluation in human beings and has been extensively tested in dogs with naturally occurring cancers [24], including its use with lomustine in a randomized placebo-controlled trial in relapsed canine lymphoma [32].

COMBINATION THERAPY APPROACHES

The most successful approaches to cancer treatment generally involve multiple forms of therapy (eg, surgery, radiation, chemotherapy); within the field of medical oncology, the use of multiple drug combinations is regarded as superior to single-agent therapy. It is not likely to be different in the new era of more targeted therapeutic approaches like inhibition of tumor angiogenesis. Even the earliest studies demonstrated improvement of metronomic chemotherapy when combined with a targeted antiangiogenic drug. Klement and colleagues [8] highlighted the utility of a combination approach targeting VEGF, which is not only a powerful proangiogenic growth factor but is a strong prosurvival factor for endothelial cells during conditions of stress (eg, exposure to chemotherapy) [33]. Thus, combination approaches that target the endothelium with chemotherapy are synergistic with drugs that target the VEGF survival pathway (eg, bevacizumab) [8]. The continuous low-dose administration strategy makes metronomic chemotherapy an attractive option for combination trials with targeted agents like bevacizumab; such trials are underway [12].

As has been case for many years with conventional cancer therapy, combination approaches may offer the best way to maximize an antiangiogenic response and delay or treat resistance. Most clinical trials performed to date use metronomic chemotherapy in combination with a targeted antiangiogenic agent; however, such agents have only recently become commercially available. Many preliminary trials incorporated more readily available putative antiangiogenic agents, such as nonsteroidal anti-inflammatory drugs, doxycycline, and thalidomide. Metronomic regimens are ultimately likely to combine multiple chemotherapy drugs with targeted anticancer agents. The optimal drugs and combinations are unknown, but effective metronomic doublet pairings (eg, cyclophosphamide with uracil plus tegafur [UFT; a fluoropyrimidine] [34–36] or methotrexate in breast cancer) have been reported [37].

CLINICAL TRIALS

The clinical trial that spawned the most interest in further evaluation of combination metronomic chemotherapy was a study evaluating the effect of daily low-dose cyclophosphamide and twice-weekly methotrexate in 64 women with progressive, advanced, and refractory breast cancer. The overall response rate in this heavily pretreated population was 32%, including 2 complete responders, 10 partial responders, and 12 patients who had stable disease lasting 6 months or longer [37,38]. In addition, favorable results have been reported involving cancers that have particular relevance to veterinarians, including non-Hodgkin's lymphoma [39], hemangiosarcoma [40,41], melanoma [42], soft tissue sarcoma [42] and prostate cancer [43,44]. Currently, several phase II clinical trials are investigating metronomic combinations against malignant glioma, non-small cell lung cancer, ovarian carcinoma, head and neck squamous cell carcinoma, renal cell carcinoma, hepatocellular carcinoma, and pancreatic carcinoma [45–47]; this list continues to grow [12]. Most of these trials combine daily oral cyclophosphamide with a commercially available targeted antiangiogenic drug (eg, bevacizumab) or a nonsteroidal anti-inflammatory drug, such as celecoxib (Celebrex). Other alkylating agents, such as trophosphamide or temozolomide, have also been popular choices in trials published thus far, and other seemingly targeted antiangiogenic drugs include thalidomide and the oral hypoglycemic agent pioglitazone.

The only veterinary clinical trials involving metronomic therapy are published as abstracts from the annual Veterinary Cancer Society conference. One study involved treatment of several different measurable tumor types (patients often had a high tumor burden) using oral cyclophosphamide at 25 mg/m^2 every other day in combination with daily oral piroxicam at 0.3 mg/kg [48]. Interim analysis identified two dogs with an objective response after 1 month of therapy. Both dogs had soft tissue sarcomas. A second trial evaluated cyclophosphamide and orally administered etoposide as adjuvant therapy for dogs with hemangiosarcoma; survival times were similar to those of dogs treated conventionally with doxorubicin [49]. There appears to be a high degree of variability in etoposide bioavailability and pharmacokinetics when that drug is administered orally to dogs, however [50]. Clearly, there is room for further optimization of these types of trials.

Finally, when compared with human MTD protocols, many would consider veterinary chemotherapeutic dosing to already be somewhat "metronomic" in nature. Doses are chosen to minimize normal tissue toxicity and combination protocols (eg, cyclophosphamide, doxorubicin, vincristine, prednisone for the treatment of lymphoma) are given at relatively tolerable doses and administered on a regular basis (often over 6 months or more), although long-term maintenance chemotherapy does not seem to offer a survival advantage over induction therapy alone [51]. A study using weekly dosing of doxorubicin at 10 mg/m^2 was less effective than the 30-mg/m^2 approach given every 3 weeks for canine lymphoma [52], however, and weekly low-dose cisplatin at 20 mg/m^2 as a radiation sensitizer resulted in unexpected myelosuppression [53]. These results illustrate the challenges facing the optimal use of chemotherapy, and it is important to keep in mind that antiangiogenic metronomic scheduling on its own is not likely to replace more intensive cytoreductive applications.

They may ultimately be used together; there is preclinical evidence to support this type of approach [54].

Like many therapies that target the growing tumor vasculature, objective results with metronomic chemotherapy may take considerable time to develop and may only manifest as sustained stable disease. In addition, like most applications of chemotherapy, the benefits of metronomic dosing may be maximized at the lowest tumor burden (eg, as adjuvant therapy), and early human clinical trials have been performed with a tumor burden that is often quite high. Interestingly, there may be a precedent for a metronomic adjuvant approach in the successful randomized phase III trial of daily low-dose oral UFT for the treatment of patients who have early-stage, resected, non-small cell lung cancer [55]. The fact that veterinary clinical trials can often be performed ethically with investigative approaches in the adjuvant setting, as evidenced by the metronomic trial in canine hemangiosarcoma, emphasizes the potential that exists to obtain meaningful clinical trial results sooner than is usually the case in human oncology.

SUMMARY

Using chemotherapy drugs as antiangiogenic agents is a new use for drugs that have been around for a long time. The favorable toxicity profile and reduced cost make low-dose continuous "metronomic" chemotherapy trials appealing, but there is still much to be learned. Challenges ahead include determination of the optimal tumor types, drugs, doses, schedules, and response monitoring (end points). Given the relative lack of toxicity to normal tissues, the design of clinical trials is likely to represent a departure from the traditional phase I dose escalation designs, and therefore requires effective biomarkers of optimal dosing. Further, the lack of objective tumor response to antiangiogenic treatments complicates the design and evaluation of phase II trials, necessitating the use of biomarkers of tumor response. The measurement of angiogenic growth factors and inhibitors and of CEPs and/or their precursors represents promising strategies in these areas [56].

References

[1] Kosarek CE, Kisseberth WC, Gallant SL, et al. Clinical evaluation of gemcitabine in dogs with spontaneously occurring malignancies. J Vet Intern Med 2005;19(1):81–6.

[2] Rassnick KM, Frimberger AE, Wood CA, et al. Evaluation of ifosfamide for treatment of various canine neoplasms. J Vet Intern Med 2000;14(3):271–6.

[3] Poirier VJ, Burgess KE, Adams WM, et al. Toxicity, dosage and efficacy of vinorelbine (Navelbine) in dogs with spontaneous neoplasia. J Vet Intern Med 2004;18(4):536–9.

[4] Moore AS, Kirk C, Cardona A. Intracavitary cisplatin chemotherapy experience with six dogs. J Vet Intern Med 1991;5(4):227–31.

[5] Jones PD, de Lormier LP, Kitchell BE, et al. Gemcitabine as a radiosensitizer for nonresectable feline oral squamous cell carcinoma. J Am Anim Hosp Assoc 2003;39(5):463–7.

[6] Hanahan DJ, Bergers G, Bergsland E. Less is more, regularly: metronomic dosing of cytotoxic drugs can target tumor angiogenesis in mice. J Clin Invest 2000;105:1045–7.

[7] Browder T, Butterfield CE, Kraling BM, et al. Antiangiogenic scheduling of chemotherapy improves efficacy against experimental drug-resistant cancer. Cancer Res 2000;60: 1878–86.

[8] Klement G, Baruchel S, Rak J, et al. Continuous low-dose therapy with vinblastine and VEGF receptor-2 antibody induces sustained tumor regression without overt toxicity. J Clin Invest 2000;105:R15–24.
[9] Skipper HE, Schabel FM, Mellet LB. Implications of biochemical, cytokinetic, pharmacologic and toxicologic relationships in the design of optimal therapeutic schedules. Cancer Chemother Rep 1970;54:431–50.
[10] Kamen BA, Rubin E, Glatstein E, et al. High-time chemotherapy or high time for low dose. J Clin Oncol 2000;18:2935–7.
[11] Kamen BA. Metronomic therapy: it makes sense and is patient friendly. J Pediatr Hematol Oncol 2005;27:571–2.
[12] Kerbel RS, Kamen BA. Antiangiogenic basis of low-dose metronomic chemotherapy. Nat Rev Cancer 2004;4:423–36.
[13] Miller KD, Sweeney CJ, Sledge GW. Redefining the target: chemotherapeutics as antiangiogenics. J Clin Oncol 2001;19:1195–206.
[14] Emmenegger U, Man S, Shaked Y, et al. A comparative analysis of low dose metronomic cyclophosphamide reveals absent or low grade toxicity on tissues highly sensitive to the toxic effects of maximum tolerated dose regimens. Cancer Res 2004;64:3994–4000.
[15] Bocci G, Nicolaou KC, Kerbel R. Protracted low-dose effects on human endothelial cell proliferation and survival in vitro reveal a selective antiangiogenic window for various chemotherapeutic drugs. Cancer Res 2002;62:6938–43.
[16] Wang J, Lou R, Lesniewski R, et al. Paclitaxel at ultra low concentrations inhibits angiogenesis without affecting cellular microtubule assembly. Anticancer Drugs 2003;14:13–9.
[17] Vacca A, Iurlaro M, Ribatti D, et al. Antiangiogenesis is produced by nontoxic doses of vinblastine. Blood 1999;94:4143–55.
[18] Asahara T, Murahara T, Sullivan A, et al. Isolation of putative progenitor endothelial cells for angiogenesis. Science 1997;275(5302):964–7.
[19] Bertolini F, Paul S, Mancuso P, et al. Maximum tolerable dose and low-dose metronomic chemotherapy have opposite effects on the mobilization and viability of circulating endothelial progenitor cells. Cancer Res 2003;63:4342–6.
[20] Man S, Bocci G, Francia G, et al. Antitumor and anti-angiogenic effects in mice of low dose (metronomic) cyclophosphamide administered continuously through the drinking water. Cancer Res 2002;62:2731–5.
[21] Shaked Y, Emmenegger U, Man S, et al. The optimal biological dose of metronomic chemotherapy regimens is associated with maximum antiangiogenic activity. Blood 2005;106:3058–61.
[22] Shaked Y, Bertolini F, Man S, et al. Genetic heterogeneity of the vasculogenic phenotype parallels angiogenesis: implications for cellular surrogate marker analysis of antiangiogenesis. Cancer Cells 2005;7:101–11.
[23] Schneider M, Tjwa M, Carmeliet P. A surrogate marker to monitor angiogenesis at last. Cancer Cells 2005;7:3–4.
[24] Rusk A, McKeegan E, Haviv F, et al. Preclinical evaluation of anti-angiogenic thrombospondin-1 peptide mimetics, ABT-526 and ABT-510, in companion dogs with naturally occurring cancers. Clin Cancer Res 2006;12(24):7444–55.
[25] Kerbel RS. Therapeutic implications of intrinsic or induced angiogenic growth factor redundancy in tumors revealed. Cancer Cells 2005;8:269–71.
[26] Rak J, Yu JL, Kerbel RS, et al. What do oncogenic mutations have to do with angiogenesis/vascular dependence of tumors? Cancer Res 2002;62(7):1931–4.
[27] Bocci G, Francia G, Man S, et al. Thombospondin-1, a mediator of the antiangiogenic effects of low-dose metronomic chemotherapy. Proc Natl Acad Sci U S A 2003;100:12917–22.
[28] Hamano Y, Sugimoto H, Soubasakos MA, et al. Thombospondin-1 associated with tumor microenvironment contributes to low-dose cyclophosphamide-mediated endothelial cell apoptosis and tumor growth suppression. Cancer Res 2004;64:1570–4.

[29] Yap R, Veliceasa D, Emmenegger U, et al. Metronomic low-dose chemotherapy boosts CD95-dependent antiangiogenic effect of the thrombospondin peptide ABT-510: a complementation antiangiogenic strategy. Clin Cancer Res 2005;11:6678–85.
[30] Kieran MW, Turner CD, Rubin JB, et al. A feasibility trial of antiangiogenic (metronomic) chemotherapy in pediatric patients with recurrent or progressive cancer. J Pediatr Hematol Oncol 2005;27(11):573–81.
[31] Damber JE, Vallbo C, Albertsson P, et al. The anti-tumor effect of low-dose continuous chemotherapy may partly be mediated by thrombospondin. Cancer Chemother Pharmacol 2006;58:354–60.
[32] Rusk A, Cozzi E, Stebbins M, et al. Cooperative activity of cytotoxic chemotherapy with antiangiogenic thrombospondin-1 peptides, ABT-526 in pet dogs with relapsed lymphoma. Clin Cancer Res 2006;12(24):7456–64.
[33] Tran J, Master Z, Yu JL, et al. A role for survivin in chemoresistance of endothelial cells mediated by VEGF. Proc Natl Acad Sci U S A 2002;99:4349–54.
[34] Ogawa Y, Ishikawa T, Chung SH, et al. Oral UFT and cyclophosphamide combination chemotherapy for metastatic breast cancer. Anticancer Res 2003;23:3453–7.
[35] Nio Y, Iguchi C, Kodama H, et al. Cyclophosphamide augments the anti-tumor efficacy of uracil and tegafur by inhibiting dihydropyrimidine dehydrogenase. Oncol Rep 2007;17:153–9.
[36] Munoz R, Man S, Shaked Y, et al. Highly efficacious non-toxic treatment for advanced metastatic breast cancer using combination UFT-cyclophosphamide metronomic chemotherapy. Cancer Res 2006;66:3386–91.
[37] Colleoni M, Rocca A, Sandri MT, et al. Low dose oral methotrexate and cyclophosphamide in metastatic breast cancer: antitumor activity and correlation with vascular endothelial growth factor levels. Ann Oncol 2002;13:73–80.
[38] Orlando L, Cardillo A, Rocca A, et al. Prolonged clinical benefit with metronomic chemotherapy in patients with metastatic breast cancer. Anticancer Drugs 2006;17:961–7.
[39] Buckstein R, Crump M, Shaked Y, et al. High dose celecoxib and metronomic "low dose" cyclophosphamide is effective and safe therapy in patients with relapsed and refractory aggressive histology NHL. Clin Cancer Res 2006;12:5190–8.
[40] Vogt T, Hafner C, Bross K, et al. Antiangiogenic therapy with pioglitazone, rofecoxib, and metronomic trofosphamide in patients with advanced malignant vascular tumors. Cancer 2003;98:2251–6.
[41] Kopp HG, Kanz L, Hartmann JT. Complete remission of relapsing high-grade angiosarcoma with single-agent metronomic trophosphamide. Anticancer Drugs 2006;17:997–8.
[42] Reichle A, Bross K, Vogt T, et al. Pioglitazone and rofecoxib combined with angiostatically scheduled trofosphamide in the treatment of far-advanced melanoma and soft tissue sarcoma. Cancer 2004;101:2247–56.
[43] Lord R, Nair S, Schache A, et al. Low dose metronomic oral cyclophosphamide for hormone resistant prostate cancer: a phase II study. J Urol 2007;177:2136–40.
[44] Glode LM, Crighton F, Barqawi A, et al. Metronomic therapy with cyclophosphamide and dexamethasone for prostate cancer. Cancer 2003;98:1643–8.
[45] Kong DS, Lee JI, Kim WS, et al. A pilot study of metronomic temozolomide treatment in patients with recurrent temozolomide-refractory glioblastoma. Oncol Rep 2006;16:1117–21.
[46] Correale P, Cerretani D, Remondo C, et al. A novel metronomic chemotherapy regimen of weekly platinum and daily oral etoposide in high-risk non-small cell lung cancer patients. Oncol Rep 2006;16:133–40.
[47] Krzyzanowska MK, Tannock IF, Lockwood G, et al. A phase II trial of continuous low-dose oral cyclophosphamide and celecoxib in patients with renal cell carcinoma. Cancer Chemother Pharmacol 2007;60:135–41.
[48] Mutsaers AJ, Mohammed SI, DeNicola DB, et al. "Metronomic" chemotherapy in veterinary oncology, a pilot study [abstract]. In: Proceedings of the 21st veterinary cancer society conference. Baton Rouge (LA), 2001. p. 41.

[49] Lana S, U'Ren L, Plaza S, et al. Comparison of continuous low-dose oral chemotherapy with conventional doxorubicin chemotherapy for adjuvant therapy of hemangiosarcoma in dogs [abstract]. In: Proceedings of the 26th veterinary cancer society conference. Pine Mountain (GA), 2006. p. 84.

[50] Flory AB, Rassnick KM, Balkman CE, et al. Bioavailability and pharmacokinetics of an oral preparation of etoposide in tumor-bearing dogs [abstract]. In: Proceedings of the 26th veterinary cancer society conference. Pine Mountain (GA), 2006. p. 29.

[51] Garrett LD, Thamm DH, Chun R, et al. Evaluation of a 6-month chemotherapy protocol with no maintenance therapy for dogs with lymphoma. J Vet Intern Med 2002;16(6):704–9.

[52] Ogilvie GK, Vail DM, Klein MK, et al. Weekly administration of low-dose doxorubicin for treatment of malignant lymphoma in dogs. J Am Vet Med Assoc 1991;198(10):1762–4.

[53] Hahn KA, Rohrbach BW, Legendre AM, et al. Hematologic changes associated with weekly low-dose cisplatin administration in dogs. Vet Clin Pathol 1997;26(1):29–31.

[54] Shaked Y, Emmenegger U, Francia G, et al. Low-dose metronomic combined with intermittent bolus-dose cyclophosphamide is an effective long-term chemotherapy treatment strategy. Cancer Res 2005;65:7045–51.

[55] Kato H, Ichinose Y, Ohta M, et al. A randomized trial of adjuvant chemotherapy with uracil-tegafur for adenocarcinoma of the lung. N Engl J Med 2004;350:1713–21.

[56] Mancuso P, Colleoni M, Calleri A, et al. Circulating endothelial cell kinetics and viability predict survival in breast cancer patients receiving metronomic chemotherapy. Blood 2006;108:452–9.

The Role of Bisphosphonates in the Management of Patients That Have Cancer

Timothy M. Fan, DVM, PhD

Department of Veterinary Clinical Medicine, University of Illinois at Urbana-Champaign, 1008 West Hazelwood Drive, Urbana, IL 61802, USA

Bisphosphonates are widely and effectively used for the management of pathologic bone resorption in people. Chemically, bisphosphonates are synthetic analogues of inorganic pyrophosphate that can inhibit calcium phosphate precipitation in vitro and biologic calcification in vivo [1]. Based on their ability to adsorb bone mineral, bisphosphonates were initially used in the detergent industry as demineralizing agents and then for diagnostic purposes in bone scanning. In the past decade, bisphosphonates have been intensely investigated as antineoplastic agents, with several bisphosphonates demonstrating use in preventing and treating skeletal complications of malignancy.

The effective treatment of bone disorders by bisphosphonates is attributed to their differential effect on bone resorption and bone mineralization. At therapeutic concentrations, bisphosphonates inhibit bone resorption without impeding the process of bone mineralization. This net effect results in stabilization and even enhancement of bone mineral density within areas of active bone remodeling. Bisphosphonates inhibit bone resorption principally through the reduction of osteoclast activities and the induction of osteoclast apoptosis [2].

Bisphosphonates have been extensively used for treating metastatic bone disease in human beings, showing effectiveness in alleviating bone pain, improving quality-of-life scores, and even providing an overall survival benefit in some studies. It is standard of care in human oncology to use bisphosphonates for treating hypercalcemia of malignancy and for the prevention of skeletal-related events (SREs), including pathologic fractures associated with metastatic bone disease. Despite the clear role of bisphosphonates for treating human patients who have cancer, their utility in companion animals that have spontaneously arising skeletal tumors requires further elucidation. Given the universal biology of malignant bone destruction, however, it is reasonable to assume that bisphosphonates are potentially effective for treating dogs and cats with

E-mail address: t-fan@uiuc.edu

bone-invasive tumors. This review discusses the fundamental properties of bisphosphonates, including pharmacology, mechanisms of action, adverse side effects, potential anticancer activities, therapeutic monitoring, and utility for treating malignant osteolysis in tumor-bearing dogs and cats.

CHEMICAL STRUCTURE AND ANTIRESORPTIVE POTENCY

Pyrophosphonates are naturally occurring compounds composed of two phosphonate groups covalently bound to a common oxygen molecule (Fig. 1A). Despite the capacity to inhibit bone resorption in vitro, natural pyrophosphonates are readily hydrolyzed by ubiquitous biologic phosphatases in vivo, and thus are clinically ineffective for managing pathologic bone resorption [2,3]. Based on the desirable in vitro characteristics yet limited in vivo effects of natural pyrophosphonates, the development of synthetic analogues with similar physicochemical properties but resistance to enzymatic hydrolysis was initiated. Substitution of the oxygen molecule with a carbon atom (geminal carbon) (Fig. 1B) created a chemical structure resistant to hydrolysis but still active as an inhibitor of bone resorption—the progenitor of the bisphosphonate drug family.

In addition to the geminal carbon atom modification, bisphosphonates contain two chains of variable structure called R_1 and R_2 groups (see Fig. 1B). Most commonly, the R_1 position is composed of a hydroxyl group, which allows for high binding affinity with calcium crystals and bone matrix. Although the R_1 group enhances binding affinity to divalent metal ions, such as calcium found in bone matrix, the relative antiresorptive potency of bisphosphonates is attributed to the chemical structure of their R_2 group (Table 1) [3]. Manipulating the R_2 group by lengthening the carbon backbone or by the insertion of a nitrogen atom dramatically increases relative antiresorptive potency [3,4]. Based on variable R_2 groups, bisphosphonates are segregated into two distinct categories. First-generation bisphosphonates (ie, non–nitrogen-containing bisphosphonates) have lesser antiresorptive activity and include etidronate (Didronel) and clodronate (Ostac). Second- and third-generation bisphosphonates (ie, aminobisphosphonates) contain a nitrogen atom within their R_2 group; are

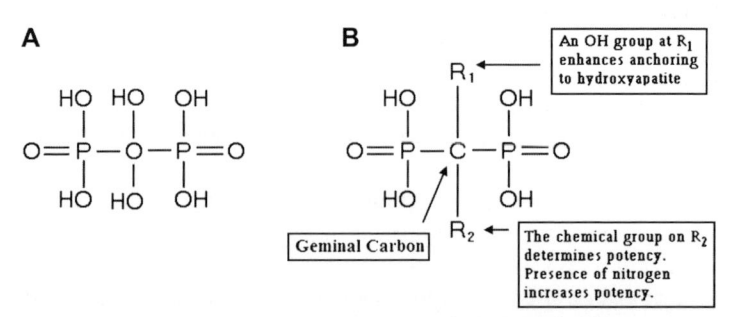

Fig. 1. General chemical structure of natural pyrophosphonates (A) and synthetic bisphosphonate structure containing geminal carbon substitution and R_1 and R_2 groups (B).

Table 1
Formulation and potency of commercially available bisphosphonates

Drug	R₁	R₂	RAP[a]	Formulation
Etidronate	OH	CH₃	1	Oral
Clodronate	Cl	Cl	10	Oral/parenteral
Tiludronate	OH	4-Chlorophenylthiomethylene	10	Oral
Pamidronate	OH	(CH₂)₂NH₂	100	Parenteral
Alendronate	OH	(CH₂)₃NH₂	1000	Oral
Risedronate	OH	Amine ring structure	5000	Oral
Ibandronate	OH	Tertiary amine	5000	Oral/parenteral
Zoledronate	OH	Amine ring structure	10,000	Parenteral

Abbreviations: Cl, chloride; OH, hydroxyl group.
[a] Relative antiresorptive potency in comparison with etidronate.

more potent inhibitors of bone resorption; and include pamidronate (Aredia), alendronate (Fosamax), risedronate (Actonel), ibandronate (Boniva), and zoledronate (Zometa).

PHARMACOKINETICS
Bisphosphonate Absorption

Bisphosphonates are commercially available as oral or intravenous formulations (see Table 1). As a drug class, the oral bioavailability of bisphosphonates is generally low (<5%) for all species evaluated, including human beings, monkeys, dogs, rats, and mice [3,5–7]. Some bisphosphonates, such as etidronate, possess low to modest intestinal absorption rates in some species, however, including dogs, which have an absorption rate of 15% to 20% [6].

After ingestion, drugs pass through the gastrointestinal (GI) lumen into the bloodstream by two principle mechanisms: transcellular migration and intercellular transport. Transcellular migration of drugs requires the movement of compounds into and through the GI epithelium before reaching systemic circulation. Intercellular transport necessitates the movement of drugs through tight junctions between adjacent epithelial cells. Physical and chemical characteristics of drugs favoring efficient transcellular or intercellular transport include high lipophilicity, small molecular size (<150 kd), low chelation capacity, and neutral charge at physiologic pH. The poor oral absorption of bisphosphonates is attributed to their low lipophilicity, relatively large molecular weight (>200 kd), high propensity to chelate biologic cations, and ionized state at physiologic pH [3].

Although bisphosphonates are poorly absorbed based on their inherent chemical characteristics, dosing regimens and patient factors may also influence oral bioavailability. First, with higher quantities administered orally, a greater than proportional increase in bisphosphonate concentration is observed in circulation and bone [5]. Mechanistically, the dose-dependent increase in bisphosphonate absorption is thought to result from the chelation of cations at the intestinal luminal surface, with the subsequent widening of epithelial tight junctions, which facilitates transcellular transport. Second, the oral absorption of bisphosphonates is dramatically influenced by the presence of food. In studies with healthy rats and human volunteers, the absorption of alendronate is increased fivefold in the fasted state [5,8,9]. Third, although the predominant sites of oral bisphosphonate absorption are the duodenum and jejunum [5], pathologic findings of the upper intestinal tract, including inflammatory conditions such as Crohn's disease, do not seem to affect, positively or negatively, oral bisphosphonate absorption [10]. As such, bisphosphonate dose modifications seem unnecessary in patients diagnosed with concurrent pathologic intestinal conditions.

Despite the low oral bioavailability of bisphosphonates, their high affinity for hydroxyapatite permits even the smallest quantities absorbed to exert bone biologic activities. Given their potent effects, one oral bisphosphonate (etidronate) and several oral aminobisphosphonates (eg, alendronate, tiludronate, risedronate, ibandronate) have all received US Food and Drug Administration (FDA) approval for the prevention and treatment of nonmalignant bone disorders in people, including osteoporosis and Paget's disease. The use of oral bisphosphonates is not approved for managing cancer-related conditions, however. Only potent intravenous aminobisphosphonates, such as pamidronate, ibandronate, and zoledronate, are approved by the FDA for the prevention and treatment of SREs (eg, hypercalcemia, pathologic fracture, spinal cord compression).

Bisphosphonate Distribution

With conventional dosing regimens, bisphosphonates are widely distributed throughout the body. With the exception of renal parenchyma, concentrations of bisphosphonates within noncalcified tissues, such as the spleen, liver, and lung, rapidly decline in parallel with circulating plasma levels. Only with extremely high intravenous dosages in rodent studies has moderate accumulation of bisphosphonates been identified in spleen, liver, and lung tissues [11–13]. Unlike noncalcified organ systems, bisphosphonates achieve high concentrations for prolonged durations within the bone matrix. Studies with oral alendronate have demonstrated prolonged half-life in bone, estimated to be 3 years for dogs and longer than 10 years for people [3,5].

Despite preferential uptake by calcified tissues, the distribution of bisphosphonates within the macroanatomic compartments of bone (cancellous versus cortical) seems to be nonuniform. Several factors account for the heterogeneous uptake of bisphosphonates within bone, including basal resorptive activity, blood flow, and surface-to-volume ratio. The fact that bisphosphonates preferentially concentrate in cancellous bone in comparison with cortical bone is confirmed by rodent and dog studies in which the concentration of bisphosphonates found within metaphyseal and epiphyseal regions of long bones is two to three times greater than that isolated from diaphyseal regions [14,15]. The differential distribution of bisphosphonates within cancellous bone is likely attributed to its higher basal resorption rate, greater blood flow, and increased surface-to-volume ratio in comparison with cortical bone. Despite avid distribution within cancellous bone, the uptake of bisphosphonates by bone seems to be saturable, because the administration of sufficiently high concentrations of bisphosphonates into circulation eventually results in a less than proportional increase in bone [15].

Bisphosphonate Metabolism, Excretion, and Terminal Elimination

As mentioned previously, bisphosphonates are resistant to phosphatase-induced hydrolysis. As a drug class, bisphosphonates have been demonstrated to be chemically stable in research animals, including dogs, rats, and monkeys [16]. Based on their physicochemical properties, they are not converted to reactive intermediates or metabolites, and therefore possess a low likelihood for untoward toxicity.

Bisphosphonates are highly water soluble, and their biliary excretion is negligible (<0.5%) [16]. Renal elimination is likely an active process, although the exact transport system involved is unknown [17], but the excretion of bisphosphonates by renal tubules is concentration dependent and saturable [16]. Therefore, administering high concentrations of bisphosphonates over short courses of time results in greater circulating plasma bisphosphonate levels and increases in bisphosphonate concentrations within calcified and noncalcified tissues.

The calculated plasma half-life of most bisphosphonates is rapid, approximately 1 to 2 hours. The short circulating half-life of bisphosphonates results from the rapid redistribution of drug to bone matrixes (nonrenal clearance) for adsorption or to kidneys for elimination. The proportion of bisphosphonate adsorbed to bone versus that eliminated by the kidneys varies among bisphosphonates and is dictated by their relative antiresorptive potencies. Although the half-life in circulation is short, the half-life of bisphosphonates adsorbed to bone is generally long and largely depends on the rate of bone turnover. Bisphosphonates within diseased bone are released more rapidly, redistributed to plasma, and, in turn, eliminated by renal excretion.

MECHANISM OF ACTION

Bone tissue contains three kinds of cells: osteoblasts, osteocytes, and osteoclasts. Osteoblasts are responsible for new bone formation, which is achieved by their active secretion of osteoid, a protein matrix that subsequently mineralizes into bone. Once osteoblasts are entrapped within an osteoid matrix, they have reduced synthetic activities and become mature osteocytes. Through a network of interconnecting processes called canaliculi, osteocytes participate in maintaining the health of bone through the continual exchange of nutrients and wastes. Osteoclasts arise from hematopoietic stem cells of monocytic-macrophage lineage (osteoclastogenesis) and are responsible for bone resorption [18]. Osteoclastogenesis requires intracellular signaling mediated by receptor activator of nuclear factor-κB (RANKL) and macrophage colony-stimulating factor (M-CSF) [19,20]. At sites of active bone resorption, osteoclasts form specialized membrane projections, called ruffled borders, that make surface contact with bone matrix. At the ruffled border, osteoclasts secrete hydrogen ions and proteolytic enzymes, resulting in bone matrix degradation and subsequent release of calcium and phosphorous [21].

The primary therapeutic effect of bisphosphonates is to reduce the rate and magnitude of pathologic bone resorption. This effect is achieved when adsorbed bisphosphonates are released from hydroxyapatite matrix during osteoclastic-mediated resorption and subsequently endocytosed by osteoclasts. The cellular uptake of bisphosphonates by osteoclasts results in the disruption of intracellular metabolism and leads to apoptosis [22,23]. Although all bisphosphonates are able to induce apoptosis of osteoclasts in vitro and in vivo, two different mechanisms of action have been identified. Non–nitrogen-containing bisphosphonates cause osteoclast apoptosis by substituting phosphate groups in the ATP molecule, yielding a nonhydrolysable cytotoxic compound [24,25]. Conversely, aminobisphosphonates induce osteoclast apoptosis by inhibiting farnesyl pyrophosphate synthase (FPPS), a key enzyme of the mevalonate pathway. Inhibition of FPPS interferes with the prenylation of small guanosine triphosphate (GTP)–binding proteins, including Ras, Rho, and Rac, resulting in aberrant intracellular signaling and subsequent osteoclast apoptosis [26].

ADVERSE EFFECTS

Orally and intravenously administered bisphosphonates are associated with low incidences of adverse side effects; the spectrum of reported toxicities is principally related to the route of drug administration. With the advent of more potent aminobisphosphonates, the quantity and frequency of drug administration required to exert bone biologic effects have been dramatically reduced; consequently, so has the incidence of most adverse effects. Despite the low incidence of side effects, unexpected and significant complications associated with bisphosphonate therapy have recently been described [27], requiring the medical oncology community to reconsider the safety of chronic antiresorptive therapies for managing pathologic bone disorders.

Gastrointestinal Adverse Events

Oral bisphosphonates (eg, clodronate, alendronate, ibandronate) are poorly absorbed from the intestinal tract and can cause diarrhea, epigastric pain, esophagitis, and esophageal ulceration [28–30]. In people with osteoporosis, oral alendronate may cause GI side effects, with erosive esophagitis comprising up to 16% of all reported adverse events [31]. The cause of esophagitis is direct chemical irritation secondary to prolonged mucosal-drug contact [31]. In addition to inadvertent retention of alendronate tablets within the esophagus, bisphosphonate-induced esophagitis may result from intermittent or partial reflux of acidic gastric contents containing bisphosphonates into the esophagus [29]. Thus, it is recommended that oral bisphosphonates be taken with adequate volumes of water and that patients refrain from lying down after ingestion to minimize the chance of gastroesophageal reflux.

Acute Systemic Inflammatory Reaction

Intravenous bisphosphonates have a modest potential to cause acute systemic inflammatory reactions characterized by fever, muscle and joint pain, nausea, vomiting, and edema [32]. In patients treated with pamidronate, zoledronate, or ibandronate, the incidence of acute systemic inflammatory reactions may approach 25% [32]. Mechanistically, systemic inflammation secondary to intravenously administered bisphosphonates is caused by elevations in circulating inflammatory cytokines, including interleukin (IL)-6 and tumor necrosis factor (TNF)-α [33–35]. The cellular source of IL-6 and TNFα is γδ T cells [36], which are activated through the recognition of aminobisphosphonates as phosphoantigens [37–39]. Acute systemic inflammatory reactions do not seem to be dose dependent and are typically self-limiting and resolve completely within 1 to 2 days after bisphosphonate infusion.

Ocular Complications

Rare adverse effects of intravenously administered bisphosphonates (<1.0%) include conjunctivitis, uveitis, scleritis, episcleritis, palpebral edema, and optic inflammation [40]. Prior clinical signs consistent with bisphosphonate-associated acute systemic inflammatory reactions seem to predispose patients to ocular complications, suggesting that ocular pathologic findings are a facet of acute systemic inflammatory reactions.

Acute and Chronic Renal Failure

Intravenous infusion of pamidronate and zoledronate has been associated with acute and chronic renal failure [41]. Of the commercially available intravenously administered formulations, zoledronate is most likely to cause renal tubule injury. The risk for renal failure is directly related to infusion duration length and total dosage, with rapid infusions of large quantities carrying the greatest risk for renal tubule injury. Predictive factors for developing zoledronate-induced renal dysfunction include patient age, cumulative number of doses, concomitant therapy with nonsteroidal anti-inflammatory drugs (NSAIDs), and current or prior treatment with cisplatin [42]. Histopathologic changes associated with kidney failure include acute tubular necrosis with loss of the brush border of the tubular cells [43]. The mechanism for acute kidney failure is speculated to be aminobisphosphonate interference with ATP-dependent metabolic pathways and damage of cytoskeletal structures within renal tubule cells [32].

Nephrotic Syndrome

Only intravenously administered pamidronate has been incriminated in the rare development of collapsing focal segmental glomerulosclerosis resulting in severe protein-losing nephropathy [44]. Electron microscopic examination of affected kidney glomeruli demonstrates hypertrophy and loss of foot processes in podocytes [45]. Given that the kidney is the only noncalcified organ that is exposed to relatively high concentrations of aminobisphosphonates after intravenous administration, it has been speculated that interference with ATP-dependent metabolic pathways is responsible for acute glomeruli damage [32].

Electrolyte Abnormalities

Treatment with intravenously administered bisphosphonates can cause hypocalcemia, hypophosphatemia, and hypomagnesemia. The most frequent abnormality after infusions with pamidronate or zoledronate is hypophosphatemia, which may occur in up to 50% of patients treated for hypercalcemia of malignancy [32]. Hypocalcemia after bisphosphonate therapy is also relatively common, with identified risk factors for its development being preexisting hypovitaminosis D, hypoparathyroidism, and hypomagnesemia [32]. Additionally, rapid rates and large concentrations of infused drug predispose to hypocalcemia.

Osteonecrosis of the Maxilla and Mandible

Several orally and intravenously administered aminobisphosphonates (eg, alendronate, risedronate, pamidronate, ibandronate, zoledronate) have been associated with osteonecrosis of the jaw (ONJ). Although many aminobisphosphonates may induce ONJ, most reported cases are associated with intravenous infusions of zoledronate and pamidronate [46,47]. The pathogenesis for ONJ remains poorly defined; however, two theories are proposed. First, ONJ may result from the profound and long-lasting osteoclastic-inhibiting effects of potent intravenously administered aminobisphosphonates, which results in the absolute cessation of necessary bone remodeling. In the absence of homeostatic bone turnover, the release of bone morphogenetic proteins and growth hormones derived from the bone matrix does not occur. Subsequently, the induction of stem cells to renew senescent osteoblasts and osteocytes is dramatically reduced. Ultimately, failure to renew the functional osteon unit results in acellular, hypovascular, and necrotic bone [48,49]. Second, ONJ may result from the antiangiogenic properties of the more potent aminobisphosphonates, which leads to the loss of nutrient blood vessels supplying the jaw bones and subsequent avascular necrosis [49]. Although bone avascularity is a hallmark of ONJ pathologic findings, more potent antiangiogenic agents, such as thalidomide, have not been associated with ONJ development. Based on these observations, the pathogenesis of ONJ is likely complex and multifactorial.

ANTICANCER MOLECULAR TARGETS

Although oral bisphosphonates are effective for the prevention and management of nonmalignant and slowly progressive bone resorptive disorders, such as osteoporosis and Paget's disease, only intravenously administered aminobisphosphonates are approved by the FDA for treating malignant osteolysis and its associated complications. By inducing osteoclast apoptosis, intravenously administered aminobisphosphonates reduce the incidence of SREs, including hypercalcemia of malignancy, pathologic fracture, and spinal cord compression. In addition to their potent antiresorptive effects, intravenously administered aminobisphosphonates demonstrate direct anticancer properties in vitro and in vivo, which provides added rational for their use in treating cancer-related bone disorders [50].

Antiproliferative Effects

By inhibiting the mevalonate pathway, aminobisphosphonates block necessary prenylation steps required for subcellular localization of signaling proteins involved in cancer cell proliferation and survival [26,51]. Apoptosis and cell cycle arrest are two in vitro mechanisms for how aminobisphosphonates may inhibit cancer growth. Aminobisphosphonates induce cancer cell apoptosis by inhibiting the localization of ras or other membrane-anchored GTP-binding proteins to the inner plasma membrane. Inappropriate subcellular localization of GTP-binding proteins disrupts downstream intracellular signals mediated by the Erk and Akt survival pathways [52]. A second growth inhibitory effect of aminobisphosphonates is the induction of cell cycle arrest. Using in vitro systems, it has been demonstrated that human cancer cells incubated with aminobisphosphonates are arrested in the G1 or S phase of the cell cycle. Blockade of cell cycle progression seems to be mediated by increased p21 and p27 expression and decreased phosphorylation of retinoblastoma protein [53,54]. Although relatively high concentrations of aminobisphosphonates (>50 mM) exert antiproliferative effects in vitro, it is uncertain if these effects are operative in patients who have cancer and are treated with intravenously administered aminobisphosphonates.

Anti-Invasive Effects

Low concentrations of aminobisphosphonates (<5 mM), insufficient to induce cancer cell apoptosis or cell cycle arrest, have been demonstrated in vitro to reduce tumor cell invasiveness, adhesion, and directional migration [50,55]. Mechanistically, aminobisphosphonates prevent appropriate subcellular localization of RhoA and its subsequent downstream signaling partners. The capacity of aminobisphosphonates to reduce tumor cell invasiveness and adhesion may result from decreased matrix metalloproteinase secretion and reduced urokinase-plasminogen activator receptor expression, respectively [50,56–58]. Given that the anti-invasive effects of aminobisphosphonates are achieved at low micromolar concentrations, it is feasible that these in vitro effects occur in human patients who have cancer and are treated with intravenously administered aminobisphosphonates. This supposition is corroborated by the clinical observation that patients who have cancer and are treated with adjuvant intravenously administered aminobisphosphonates are less likely to develop additional skeletal metastases, a process requiring tumor cells to invade, adhere, and migrate successfully [59–61].

Antiangiogenesis

Of the potent intravenously administered aminobisphosphonates, zoledronate has been most intensively studied for its potential antiangiogenic properties. In vitro, zoledronate has been demonstrated to inhibit the mitogen-induced proliferation of human umbilical vein endothelial cells [62]. Additionally, zoledronate inhibits endothelial cell adhesion and migration through the downregulation of a_vb_3 integrin expression [63]. In murine models, zoledronate inhibits angiogenesis induced by basic fibroblast growth factor–impregnated implants [62] and murine myeloma-induced angiogenesis [64]. Significantly, in human patients who have cancer, concentrations of circulating angiogenic peptides, including vascular endothelial growth factor (VEGF), have been transiently yet significantly reduced after treatment with intravenously administered zoledronate [65–67]. Although zoledronate seems to reduce circulating angiogenic peptides in human patients who have cancer, it has yet to be determined if these reductions are clinically relevant for delaying the growth of primary and metastatic cancers.

THERAPEUTIC RESPONSE ASSESSMENT IN PATIENTS WHO HAVE CANCER

Unlike traditional cytotoxic agents, in which therapeutic activities are substantiated by a measurable reduction in tumor burden, assessing the biologic effectiveness of bisphosphonates for the management of malignant osteolysis is more difficult. Although self-reported decreases in bone pain can be a useful clinical indicator of therapeutic response in people, this subjective method of assessment is not possible for cancer-bearing dogs and cats. Because bisphosphonate therapy has become a cornerstone of therapy in people with skeletal metastases, newer and more accurate measures for assessing their bone biologic effects have been developed and include objective radiologic and bone-specific biochemical methodologies.

Traditional Radiologic Methods

Conventional methods for assessing the response of bone metastases to bisphosphonate therapy include plain radiography and qualitative bone scintigraphy. One limitation of plain radiographs is their insensitivity for identifying small or early bone lesions [68,69]. Furthermore, in patients who have cancer and are treated with bisphosphonates for malignant osteolysis, demonstrable radiographic changes are often delayed. Therefore, radiographic evidence of response does not represent real-time changes induced by antiresorptive therapies. Although qualitative bone scintigraphy is more sensitive than radiographs, it lacks specificity and anatomic detail [68,69]. Additionally, because bone-seeking isotopes preferentially home to skeletal sites with increased osteoblastic activities and blood flow, qualitative scintigraphy cannot distinguish between bone healing and disease progression [70].

Newer Radiologic Methods

Several imaging modalities with utility for monitoring patients who have cancer and are treated with bisphosphonates include quantitative bone scintigraphy, CT, MRI, dual-energy x-ray absorptiometry (DEXA), and positron emission tomography (PET). Quantitative bone scintigraphy correlates with disease prognosis in men diagnosed with skeletal metastases; however, serial imaging studies are time-consuming and operator dependent [71]. CT scans provide high-detail skeletal images, but scanning large anatomic regions is impractical for assessing patients who have multifocal or diffuse skeletal lesions. MRI can accurately detect changes associated with response to bisphosphonate therapy and disease progression [72]; however, MRI is costly, thus precluding its use for routine procedures. Serial scanning with DEXA is a safe procedure routinely used for assessing bone mineral density in postmenopausal women diagnosed with osteoporosis. Similarly, DEXA has proved useful for assessing changes in density of bone metastatic lesions associated with prostate and breast carcinoma. For predominantly lytic skeletal lesions, increases in mineral density at metastatic bone sites correlate with biologic response to effective anticancer and antiresorptive agents [73–76]. PET is increasingly being used to stage patients who have cancer. Based on the higher metabolic activity of cancer cells, preferential uptake of PET tracers allows for lesion identification and localization. The PET tracer F^{18} is fairly bone specific. Given that PET scans are not only sensitive but provide good spatial resolution, their increasingly routine use is likely to be beneficial for monitoring responses to bisphosphonate therapy.

Bone-Specific Biochemical Methodologies

Specific markers of bone turnover can be used to assess therapeutic response in patients who have malignant osteolysis. Under homeostatic conditions, continual remodeling of the skeleton occurs throughout life by means of the balanced coupling of osteoblastic bone deposition and osteoclastic bone resorption. During malignant osteolysis, cancer cells promote excessive osteoclastic activities, resulting in the dysregulated breakdown of bone matrix and the release of type I collagen byproducts into systemic circulation. In response to pathologic bone resorption, neighboring osteoblasts attempt a reparative process, resulting in the liberation of procollagen synthesis byproducts [71]. Byproducts of bone resorption and formation may be quantified in urine and serum and have the advantage of assessing the magnitude and directionality of bone turnover in real-time.

Although conventional bone formation markers have been evaluated in men with osteoblastic skeletal metastases responsive to bisphosphonate therapy [77], most clinical studies have investigated the utility of bone resorption markers as surrogate indices of therapeutic response. Useful bone resorption markers include collagen-pyridinium cross-links (pyridinoline and deoxypyridinoline) and type I collagen telopeptides. Type I collagen is the main structural protein of mineralized bone and accounts for approximately 90% of its organic matrix. During pathologic bone resorption, osteoclasts enzymatically degrade bone matrix, releasing amino and carboxy terminal–derived fragments of type I collagen designated as N-terminal telopeptide (NTx) and C-terminal telopeptide (CTx), respectively. These end products of bone resorption circulate in blood and, ultimately, are excreted intact in the urine. Although several bone resorption markers have been identified, urine NTx is considered to be the most accurate marker of bone resorption in human patients who have pathologic skeletal disorders [78–80]. In human patients undergoing antiresorptive therapy for such conditions as osteoporosis or malignant osteolysis, the evaluation of serial urine NTx levels can provide a sensitive and objective method to assess and monitor clinical response [81,82].

AMINOBISPHONATES IN CANCER-BEARING DOGS AND CATS

Cats and dogs with bone-invasive tumors may initially be presented for clinical signs attributable to pain and hypercalcemia of malignancy. In dogs, neoplasms commonly associated with malignant osteolysis or hypercalcemia include appendicular osteosarcoma (OSA); multiple myeloma; and metastatic carcinomas arising from prostate, mammary, urinary bladder, and apocrine gland anal sac tissues [83,84]. In cats, oral squamous cell carcinoma (OSCC) accounts for approximately 75% of malignancies involving the feline oral cavity [85] and can invade the mandibular or maxillary bones, causing malignant osteolysis, pain, and hypercalcemia [86–89]. Although tumor types vary, the mechanisms responsible for malignant skeletal destruction and bone cancer pain are similar among human beings, dogs, and cats [90]. Within the bone tumor microenvironment, cancer cells subvert osteoclast activities and promote excessive bone matrix erosion. Pathologic bone resorption by osteoclasts and production of inflammatory peptides by tumor cells stimulate the nociceptor-rich endosteum and periosteum, creating sensations of pain [91]. Given that malignant bone resorption is linked to the generation of pain [91–93], it is reasonable to believe that inhibiting bone resorption with potent intravenously administered bisphosphonates would have the potential of alleviating skeletal pain in tumor-bearing dogs and cats [91–93].

Management of Osteolytic Bone Pain

Given the prevalence of primary and metastatic bone tumors that affect veterinary patients, potent aminobisphosphonates may have a role in an adjuvant setting for the management of cancer-induced bone pain. The first reported description in the veterinary literature was the use of oral alendronate for the palliative management of 2 dogs that had OSA [94]. Based on the unexpectedly long survival times reported in this anecdotal study, the these investigators suggested that aminobisphosphonate therapy may have a role in managing canine malignant bone disorders. Given the low oral bioavailability of alendronate in dogs [16] and the sole use of intravenously administered aminobisphosphonates for the treatment of malignant osteolysis in human patients who have cancer, a prospective study principally evaluating the safety of intravenously administered pamidronate was conducted in 33 dogs diagnosed with primary and secondary skeletal tumors [95]. Intravenous pamidronate (1.0 mg/kg diluted with 0.9% sodium chloride to a total volume of 250 mL) given as a 2-hour constant rate infusion (CRI) every 28 days was well tolerated. In a subset of OSA-bearing dogs, bone biologic and clinically relevant therapeutic effects were documented as significant reductions in urine NTx concentrations, increases in relative primary tumor bone mineral density (rBMD), and subjective pain alleviation [95].

After the established safety of intravenously administered pamidronate in dogs with primary and secondary skeletal tumors, a second study consisting of 43 dogs with appendicular OSA treated with intravenously administered pamidronate (comparing 1.0 mg/kg versus 2.0 mg/kg) was conducted [96]. Although the two different doses of pamidronate did not demonstrate differences for pain alleviation, reductions in urine NTx concentrations, or increases in rBMD, there was a strong (although not significant) biologic trend for higher doses of pamidronate (2.0 mg/kg) to exert greater bone biologic effects, as reflected by larger absolute reductions in urine NTx concentrations. Overall, 12 (28%) of 43 OSA-bearing dogs treated with single-agent intravenously administered pamidronate achieved pain alleviation for longer than 4 months. In addition to the subjective analgesic effects of pamidronate reported by pet owners, changes in urine NTx concentrations and DEXA-assessed rBMD correlated with therapeutic response. These findings are highly significant because they validate the use of biochemical and radiologic surrogate indices of bone turnover for monitoring response to aminobisphosphonate therapy in bone cancer–bearing dogs.

In human patients who have cancer, intravenously administered aminobisphosphonates are often used in combination with locoregional radiotherapy, systemic chemotherapy, and oral analgesic drugs. In dogs with appendicular OSA, one study has described the bone biologic effects of combining intravenously administered pamidronate (2.0 mg/kg as a 2-hour CRI every 28 days), palliative radiotherapy (8 Gy/wk for 4 weeks), doxorubicin (30 mg/m^2 every 21 days), and oral deracoxib (1–2 mg/kg/d) for managing focal malignant osteolysis [97]. Circulating urine NTx concentrations dramatically and consistently decreased in all dogs treated, indicating that multimodality therapy inclusive of intravenously administered pamidronate exerts bone biologic effects. Additionally, all tumor-bearing dogs experienced subjective pain alleviation of variable duration, supporting the notion that intravenously administered pamidronate can be effectively combined with traditional palliative treatment options for managing dogs with appendicular OSA.

Other potent intravenously administered aminobisphosphonates for managing malignant bone pain have also been evaluated in dogs and cats. Zoledronate possesses 100-fold greater antiresorptive potency in comparison with pamidronate and has the advantage of being safely administered over a shorter period than other aminobisphosphonates. In a recent study conducted in cats diagnosed with bone-invasive OSCC, intravenously administered zoledronate dosed at 0.2 mg/kg as a 15-minute CRI every 21 to 28 days was well tolerated and exerted significant antiresorptive and antiangiogenic effects [98]. In this study, as determined by elevated basal concentrations of serum CTx, cats with bone-invasive OSCC had greater bone resorption than healthy controls. After the administration of zoledronate, cats with OSCC demonstrated significant reductions in serum CTx and soluble vascular endothelial growth factor (sVEGF). These findings corroborate the results from human studies, which have shown not only beneficial bone biologic activities but antiangiogenic effects subsequent to intravenously administered zoledronate [65–67].

The bone biologic effects of intravenously administered zoledronate have also been evaluated in dogs diagnosed with primary and secondary skeletal tumors [99]. In this study, zoledronate was administered at a dose of 0.25 mg/kg as a 15-minute CRI every 28 days, a treatment regimen previously demonstrated to exert bone biologic effects in healthy dogs [100]. Intravenously administered zoledronate was well tolerated, with no overt biochemical evidence of renal toxicity in patients receiving multiple monthly infusions. All tumor-bearing dogs demonstrated dramatic and significant reductions in urine NTx concentrations after therapy, indicating that zoledronate exerts potent global antiresorptive effects. Furthermore, in a subset of dogs with primary appendicular OSA (n = 10), patients achieving pain alleviation also demonstrated significant increases in rBMD. The observation for increased rBMD in conjunction with pain alleviation suggests that zoledronate inhibits local malignant osteolysis and the generation of pain within the immediate bone-tumor microenvironment.

Management of Tumor-Induced Hypercalcemia

Excessive stimulation of osteoclast-mediated bone resorption and enhanced renal tubular calcium reabsorption are the two underlying mechanisms for tumor-induced hypercalcemia. By secreting various soluble factors, including TNFβ and IL-1β [101,102], tumor cells are able to uncouple the balanced relation between bone resorption and bone formation. Similarly, the tumor-secreted factor parathyroid hormone–related peptide (PTH-rp) not only promotes osteoclastic bone resorption but enhances renal tubular calcium reabsorption [5].

Bisphosphonates reduce the magnitude of hypercalcemia by inducing osteoclast apoptosis. This results in diminished bone resorption with subsequent reductions in serum calcium levels. Despite the inhibitory effects of bisphosphonates on osteoclast-mediated hypercalcemia, they demonstrate limited effectiveness for managing hypercalcemia mediated by enhanced renal tubular calcium reabsorption [103,104]. For this reason, hypercalcemic patients with greater elevations in PTH-rp respond less favorably to bisphosphonate therapy than do hypercalcemic patients with lower levels of PTH-rp [105].

Although effective for managing tumor-induced hypercalcemia in human patients who have cancer, the use of bisphosphonates to reduce serum calcium concentrations in tumor-bearing dogs and cats is poorly documented. Only three studies have anecdotally described the use of intravenously administered pamidronate for managing hypercalcemia of malignancy identified in dogs and cats [95,106,107]. Unfortunately, none of these studies were designed to evaluate the effectiveness of single-agent pamidronate for managing hypercalcemia, because patients were treated with concurrent supportive measures, including saline-induced diuresis and calcium-wasting diuretics. Based on these limitations, it is not possible to determine if single-agent intravenously administered pamidronate is truly effective for managing malignant hypercalcemia in tumor-bearing dogs and cats. Given that most veterinary patients that have cancer manifest with hypercalcemia secondary to excessive PTH-rp production and not severe osteolysis, the effective use of pamidronate alone for treating tumor-induced hypercalcemia may be limited. If bisphosphonates are used to manage PTH-rp–mediated hypercalcemia, adjunctive use of other drugs capable of diminishing renal tubular calcium reabsorption (eg, glucocorticoids, loop diuretics) should be considered to maximize the likelihood for achieving normocalcemia.

In conclusion, bisphosphonates are effective agents for preventing and treating malignant consequences of skeletal neoplasms. Bisphosphonates inhibit bone resorption by inducing osteoclast apoptosis and may possess direct anticancer activities. As a class of drugs, bisphosphonates are not metabolized; therefore, they are rarely associated with life-threatening adverse effects. Monitoring response to bisphosphonate therapy may be accomplished through the combined use of radiologic and biochemical surrogate indices of bone metabolism. Given the shared biology in people and companion animals for the processes involved in cancer-induced osteolysis, bisphosphonate use is expected to become widely accepted for treating dogs and cats diagnosed with skeletal tumors. With their appropriate adjuvant use, bisphosphonates can provide an additional and effective treatment option for decreasing bone cancer–related pain in companion animals that have malignant osteolysis.

References

[1] Fleisch H. Bisphosphonates. Pharmacology and use in the treatment of tumour-induced hypercalcaemic and metastatic bone disease. Drugs 1991;42(6):919–44.
[2] Body JJ. Bisphosphonates. Eur J Cancer 1998;34(2):263–9.
[3] Lin JH. Bisphosphonates: a review of their pharmacokinetic properties. Bone 1996;18(2): 75–85.
[4] Shinoda H, Adamek G, Felix R, et al. Structure-activity relationships of various bisphosphonates. Calcif Tissue Int 1983;35(1):87–99.
[5] Grill V, Ho P, Body JJ, et al. Parathyroid hormone-related protein: elevated levels in both humoral hypercalcemia of malignancy and hypercalcemia complicating metastatic breast cancer. J Clin Endocrinol Metab 1991;73(6):1309–15.
[6] Michael WR, King WR, Wakim JM. Metabolism of disodium ethane-1-hydroxy-1,1-diphosphonate (disodium etidronate) in the rat, rabbit, dog and monkey. Toxicol Appl Pharmacol 1972;21(4):503–15.
[7] Barrett J, Worth E, Bauss F, et al. Ibandronate: a clinical pharmacological and pharmacokinetic update. J Clin Pharmacol 2004;44(9):951–65.
[8] Gertz BJ, Holland SD, Kline WF, et al. Studies of the oral bioavailability of alendronate. Clin Pharmacol Ther 1995;58(3):288–98.
[9] Porras AG, Holland SD, Gertz BJ. Pharmacokinetics of alendronate. Clin Pharmacokinet 1999;36(5):315–28.
[10] Cremers SC, van Hogezand R, Banffer D, et al. Absorption of the oral bisphosphonate alendronate in osteoporotic patients with Crohn's disease. Osteoporos Int 2005;16(12): 1727–30.
[11] Monkkonen J, Koponen HM, Ylitalo P. Comparison of the distribution of three bisphosphonates in mice. Pharmacol Toxicol 1990;66(4):294–8.

[12] Monkkonen J, van Rooijen N, Ylitalo P. Effects of clodronate and pamidronate on splenic and hepatic phagocytic cells of mice. Pharmacol Toxicol 1991;68(4):284-6.
[13] Monkkonen J, Ylitalo P. The tissue distribution of clodronate (dichloromethylene bisphosphonate) in mice. The effects of vehicle and the route of administration. Eur J Drug Metab Pharmacokinet 1990;15(3):239-43.
[14] Kasting GB, Francis MD. Retention of etidronate in human, dog, and rat. J Bone Miner Res 1992;7(5):513-22.
[15] Lin JH, Chen IW, Duggan DE. Effects of dose, sex, and age on the disposition of alendronate, a potent antiosteolytic bisphosphonate, in rats. Drug Metab Dispos 1992;20(4):473-8.
[16] Lin JH, Duggan DE, Chen IW, et al. Physiological disposition of alendronate, a potent antiosteolytic bisphosphonate, in laboratory animals. Drug Metab Dispos 1991;19(5):926-32.
[17] Lin JH, Chen IW, Deluna FA, et al. Renal handling of alendronate in rats. An uncharacterized renal transport system. Drug Metab Dispos 1992;20(4):608-13.
[18] Marks SC Jr, Walker DG. The hematogenous origin of osteoclasts: experimental evidence from osteopetrotic (microphthalmic) mice treated with spleen cells from beige mouse donors. Am J Anat 1981;161(1):1-10.
[19] Nakagawa N, Kinosaki M, Yamaguchi K, et al. RANK is the essential signaling receptor for osteoclast differentiation factor in osteoclastogenesis. Biochem Biophys Res Commun 1998;253(2):395-400.
[20] Tsurukai T, Udagawa N, Matsuzaki K, et al. Roles of macrophage-colony stimulating factor and osteoclast differentiation factor in osteoclastogenesis. J Bone Miner Metab 2000;18(4):177-84.
[21] Holtrop ME, King GJ. The ultrastructure of the osteoclast and its functional implications. Clin Orthop Relat Res 1977;123:177-96.
[22] Hughes DE, Wright KR, Uy HL, et al. Bisphosphonates promote apoptosis in murine osteoclasts in vitro and in vivo. J Bone Miner Res 1995;10(10):1478-87.
[23] Selander KS, Monkkonen J, Karhukorpi EK, et al. Characteristics of clodronate-induced apoptosis in osteoclasts and macrophages. Mol Pharmacol 1996;50(5):1127-38.
[24] Rodan GA. Mechanisms of action of bisphosphonates. Annu Rev Pharmacol Toxicol 1998;38:375-88.
[25] Rogers MJ, Gordon S, Benford HL, et al. Cellular and molecular mechanisms of action of bisphosphonates. Cancer 2000;88(12 Suppl):2961-78.
[26] Luckman SP, Hughes DE, Coxon FP, et al. Nitrogen-containing bisphosphonates inhibit the mevalonate pathway and prevent post-translational prenylation of GTP-binding proteins, including Ras. J Bone Miner Res 1998;13(4):581-9.
[27] Migliorati CA, Siegel MA, Elting LS. Bisphosphonate-associated osteonecrosis: a long-term complication of bisphosphonate treatment. Lancet Oncol 2006;7(6):508-14.
[28] Abraham SC, Cruz-Correa M, Lee LA, et al. Alendronate-associated esophageal injury: pathologic and endoscopic features. Mod Pathol 1999;12(12):1152-7.
[29] Adami S, Zamberlan N. Adverse effects of bisphosphonates. A comparative review. Drug Saf 1996;14(3):158-70.
[30] Body JJ. Dosing regimens and main adverse events of bisphosphonates. Semin Oncol 2001;28(4 Suppl 11):49-53.
[31] de Groen PC, Lubbe DF, Hirsch LJ, et al. Esophagitis associated with the use of alendronate. N Engl J Med 1996;335(14):1016-21.
[32] Tanvetyanon T, Stiff PJ. Management of the adverse effects associated with IV bisphosphonates. Ann Oncol 2006;17(6):897-907.
[33] Sauty A, Pecherstorfer M, Zimmer-Roth I, et al. Interleukin-6 and tumor necrosis factor alpha levels after bisphosphonates treatment in vitro and in patients with malignancy. Bone 1996;18(2):133-9.

[34] Dicuonzo G, Vincenzi B, Santini D, et al. Fever after zoledronic acid administration is due to increase in TNF-alpha and IL-6. J Interferon Cytokine Res 2003;23(11):649–54.
[35] Thiebaud D, Sauty A, Burckhardt P, et al. An in vitro and in vivo study of cytokines in the acute-phase response associated with bisphosphonates. Calcif Tissue Int 1997;61(5): 386–92.
[36] Hewitt RE, Lissina A, Green AE, et al. The bisphosphonate acute phase response: rapid and copious production of proinflammatory cytokines by peripheral blood gd T cells in response to aminobisphosphonates is inhibited by statins. Clin Exp Immunol 2005;139(1):101–11.
[37] Miyagawa F, Tanaka Y, Yamashita S, et al. Essential requirement of antigen presentation by monocyte lineage cells for the activation of primary human gamma delta T cells by aminobisphosphonate antigen. J Immunol 2001;166(9):5508–14.
[38] Das H, Wang L, Kamath A, et al. Vgamma2Vdelta2 T-cell receptor-mediated recognition of aminobisphosphonates. Blood 2001;98(5):1616–8.
[39] Dieli F, Gebbia N, Poccia F, et al. Induction of gammadelta T-lymphocyte effector functions by bisphosphonate zoledronic acid in cancer patients in vivo. Blood 2003;102(6): 2310–1.
[40] Fraunfelder FW, Fraunfelder FT, Jensvold B. Scleritis and other ocular side effects associated with pamidronate disodium. Am J Ophthalmol 2003;135(2):219–22.
[41] Body JJ, Pfister T, Bauss F. Preclinical perspectives on bisphosphonate renal safety. Oncologist 2005;10(Suppl 1):3–7.
[42] McDermott RS, Kloth DD, Wang H, et al. Impact of zoledronic acid on renal function in patients with cancer: clinical significance and development of a predictive model. J Support Oncol 2006;4(10):524–9.
[43] Markowitz GS, Fine PL, Stack JI, et al. Toxic acute tubular necrosis following treatment with zoledronate (Zometa). Kidney Int 2003;64(1):281–9.
[44] Markowitz GS, Appel GB, Fine PL, et al. Collapsing focal segmental glomerulosclerosis following treatment with high-dose pamidronate. J Am Soc Nephrol 2001;12(6): 1164–72.
[45] Barri YM, Munshi NC, Sukumalchantra S, et al. Podocyte injury associated glomerulopathies induced by pamidronate. Kidney Int 2004;65(2):634–41.
[46] Marx RE. Pamidronate (Aredia) and zoledronate (Zometa) induced avascular necrosis of the jaws: a growing epidemic. J Oral Maxillofac Surg 2003;61(9):1115–7.
[47] Farrugia MC, Summerlin DJ, Krowiak E, et al. Osteonecrosis of the mandible or maxilla associated with the use of new generation bisphosphonates. Laryngoscope 2006;116(1):115–20.
[48] Hewitt C, Farah CS. Bisphosphonate-related osteonecrosis of the jaws: a comprehensive review. J Oral Pathol Med 2007;36(6):319–28.
[49] Marx RE, Sawatari Y, Fortin M, et al. Bisphosphonate-induced exposed bone (osteonecrosis/osteopetrosis) of the jaws: risk factors, recognition, prevention, and treatment. J Oral Maxillofac Surg 2005;63(11):1567–75.
[50] Caraglia M, Santini D, Marra M, et al. Emerging anti-cancer molecular mechanisms of aminobisphosphonates. Endocr Relat Cancer 2006;13(1):7–26.
[51] Coxon FP, Helfrich MH, Larijani B, et al. Identification of a novel phosphonocarboxylate inhibitor of Rab geranylgeranyl transferase that specifically prevents Rab prenylation in osteoclasts and macrophages. J Biol Chem 2001;276(51):48213–22.
[52] Caraglia M, D'Alessandro AM, Marra M, et al. The farnesyl transferase inhibitor R115777 (Zarnestra) synergistically enhances growth inhibition and apoptosis induced on epidermoid cancer cells by zoledronic acid (Zometa) and pamidronate. Oncogene 2004;23(41):6900–13.
[53] Corey E, Brown LG, Quinn JE, et al. Zoledronic acid exhibits inhibitory effects on osteoblastic and osteolytic metastases of prostate cancer. Clin Cancer Res 2003;9(1):295–306.

[54] Reszka AA, Halasy-Nagy J, Rodan GA. Nitrogen-bisphosphonates block retinoblastoma phosphorylation and cell growth by inhibiting the cholesterol biosynthetic pathway in a keratinocyte model for esophageal irritation. Mol Pharmacol 2001;59(2):193–202.
[55] Denoyelle C, Hong L, Vannier JP, et al. New insights into the actions of bisphosphonate zoledronic acid in breast cancer cells by dual RhoA-dependent and -independent effects. Br J Cancer 2003;88(10):1631–40.
[56] Montague R, Hart CA, George NJ, et al. Differential inhibition of invasion and proliferation by bisphosphonates: anti-metastatic potential of zoledronic acid in prostate cancer. Eur Urol 2004;46(3):389–401 [discussion: 401–2].
[57] Heikkila P, Teronen O, Moilanen M, et al. Bisphosphonates inhibit stromelysin-1 (MMP-3), matrix metalloelastase (MMP-12), collagenase-3 (MMP-13) and enamelysin (MMP-20), but not urokinase-type plasminogen activator, and diminish invasion and migration of human malignant and endothelial cell lines. Anticancer Drugs 2002;13(3):245–54.
[58] Giraudo E, Inoue M, Hanahan D. An amino-bisphosphonate targets MMP-9-expressing macrophages and angiogenesis to impair cervical carcinogenesis. J Clin Invest 2004;114(5):623–33.
[59] Mystakidou K, Katsouda E, Parpa E, et al. Randomized, open label, prospective study on the effect of zoledronic acid on the prevention of bone metastases in patients with recurrent solid tumors that did not present with bone metastases at baseline. Med Oncol 2005;22(2):195–201.
[60] Diel IJ, Solomayer EF, Costa SD, et al. Reduction in new metastases in breast cancer with adjuvant clodronate treatment. N Engl J Med 1998;339(6):357–63.
[61] Leto G, Badalamenti G, Arcara C, et al. Effects of zoledronic acid on proteinase plasma levels in patients with bone metastases. Anticancer Res 2006;26(1A):23–6.
[62] Wood J, Bonjean K, Ruetz S, et al. Novel antiangiogenic effects of the bisphosphonate compound zoledronic acid. J Pharmacol Exp Ther 2002;302(3):1055–61.
[63] Bellahcene A, Chaplet M, Bonjean K, et al. Zoledronate inhibits alphavbeta3 and alphavbeta5 integrin cell surface expression in endothelial cells. Endothelium 2007;14(2):123–30.
[64] Croucher PI, De Hendrik R, Perry MJ, et al. Zoledronic acid treatment of 5T2MM-bearing mice inhibits the development of myeloma bone disease: evidence for decreased osteolysis, tumor burden and angiogenesis, and increased survival. J Bone Miner Res 2003;18(3):482–92.
[65] Ferretti G, Fabi A, Carlini P, et al. Zoledronic-acid-induced circulating level modifications of angiogenic factors, metalloproteinases and proinflammatory cytokines in metastatic breast cancer patients. Oncology 2005;69(1):35–43.
[66] Santini D, Vincenzi B, Dicuonzo G, et al. Zoledronic acid induces significant and long-lasting modifications of circulating angiogenic factors in cancer patients. Clin Cancer Res 2003;9(8):2893–7.
[67] Vincenzi B, Santini D, Dicuonzo G, et al. Zoledronic acid-related angiogenesis modifications and survival in advanced breast cancer patients. J Interferon Cytokine Res 2005;25(3):144–51.
[68] Wahner HW, Dunn WL, Riggs BL. Assessment of bone mineral. Part 2. J Nucl Med 1984;25(11):1241–53.
[69] Wahner HW, Dunn WL, Riggs BL. Assessment of bone mineral. Part 1. J Nucl Med 1984;25(10):1134–41.
[70] Janicek MJ, Hayes DF, Kaplan WD. Healing flare in skeletal metastases from breast cancer. Radiology 1994;192(1):201–4.
[71] Clamp A, Danson S, Nguyen H, et al. Assessment of therapeutic response in patients with metastatic bone disease. Lancet Oncol 2004;5(10):607–16.
[72] Frank JA, Ling A, Patronas NJ, et al. Detection of malignant bone tumors: MR imaging vs scintigraphy. AJR Am J Roentgenol 1990;155(5):1043–8.

[73] Shapiro CL, Keating J, Angell JE, et al. Monitoring therapeutic response in skeletal metastases using dual-energy x-ray absorptiometry: a prospective feasibility study in breast cancer patients. Cancer Invest 1999;17(8):566–74.
[74] Berruti A, Dogliotti L, Osella G, et al. Evaluation by dual energy X-ray absorptiometry of changed bone density in metastatic bone sites as a consequence of systemic treatment. Oncol Rep 2000;7(4):777–81.
[75] Smith GL, Doherty AP, Banks LM, et al. Dual x-ray absorptiometry detects disease- and treatment-related alterations of bone density in prostate cancer patients. Clin Exp Metastasis 2000;18(5):385–90.
[76] Koeberle D, Bacchus L, Thuerlimann B, et al. Pamidronate treatment in patients with malignant osteolytic bone disease and pain: a prospective randomized double-blind trial. Support Care Cancer 1999;7(1):21–7.
[77] Koizumi M, Yonese J, Fukui I, et al. Metabolic gaps in bone formation may be a novel marker to monitor the osseous metastasis of prostate cancer. J Urol 2002;167(4): 1863–6.
[78] Demers LM, Costa L, Lipton A. Biochemical markers and skeletal metastases. Cancer 2000;88(12 Suppl):2919–26.
[79] Lipton A, Demers L, Curley E, et al. Markers of bone resorption in patients treated with pamidronate. Eur J Cancer 1998;34(13):2021–6.
[80] Costa L, Demers LM, Gouveia-Oliveira A, et al. Prospective evaluation of the peptide-bound collagen type I cross-links N-telopeptide and C-telopeptide in predicting bone metastases status. J Clin Oncol 2002;20(3):850–6.
[81] Hanson DA, Weis MA, Bollen AM, et al. A specific immunoassay for monitoring human bone resorption: quantitation of type I collagen cross-linked N-telopeptides in urine. J Bone Miner Res 1992;7(11):1251–8.
[82] Worsfold M, Powell DE, Jones TJ, et al. Assessment of urinary bone markers for monitoring treatment of osteoporosis. Clin Chem 2004;50(12):2263–70.
[83] Rosol TJ, Nagode LA, Couto CG, et al. Parathyroid hormone (PTH)-related protein, PTH, and 1,25-dihydroxyvitamin D in dogs with cancer-associated hypercalcemia. Endocrinology 1992;131(3):1157–64.
[84] Williams LE, Gliatto JM, Dodge RK, et al. Carcinoma of the apocrine glands of the anal sac in dogs: 113 cases (1985–1995). J Am Vet Med Assoc 2003;223(6):825–31.
[85] Klein MK. Multimodality therapy for head and neck cancer. Vet Clin North Am Small Anim Pract 2003;33(3):615–28.
[86] Stebbins KE, Morse CC, Goldschmidt MH. Feline oral neoplasia: a ten-year survey. Vet Pathol 1989;26(2):121–8.
[87] Quigley PJ, Leedale AH. Tumors involving bone in the domestic cat: a review of fifty-eight cases. Vet Pathol 1983;20(6):670–86.
[88] Klausner JS, Bell FW, Hayden DW, et al. Hypercalcemia in two cats with squamous cell carcinomas. J Am Vet Med Assoc 1990;196(1):103–5.
[89] Savary KC, Price GS, Vaden SL. Hypercalcemia in cats: a retrospective study of 71 cases (1991-1997). J Vet Intern Med 2000;14(2):184–9.
[90] Barger AM, Fan TM, de Lorimier LP, et al. Expression of receptor activator of nuclear factor kappa-B ligand (RANKL) in neoplasms of dogs and cats. J Vet Intern Med 2007;21(1): 133–40.
[91] Clohisy DR, Mantyh PW. Bone cancer pain. Cancer 2003;97(3 Suppl):866–73.
[92] Goblirsch MJ, Zwolak P, Clohisy DR. Advances in understanding bone cancer pain. J Cell Biochem 2005;96(4):682–8.
[93] Luger NM, Honore P, Sabino MA, et al. Osteoprotegerin diminishes advanced bone cancer pain. Cancer Res 2001;61(10):4038–47.
[94] Tomlin JL, Sturgeon C, Pead MJ, et al. Use of the bisphosphonate drug alendronate for palliative management of osteosarcoma in two dogs. Vet Rec 2000;147(5):129–32.

[95] Fan TM, de Lorimier LP, Charney SC, et al. Evaluation of IV pamidronate administration in 33 cancer-bearing dogs with primary or secondary bone involvement. J Vet Intern Med 2005;19(1):74–80.
[96] Fan TM, de Lorimier LP, O'Dell-Anderson K, et al. Single-agent pamidronate for palliative therapy of canine appendicular osteosarcoma bone pain. J Vet Intern Med 2007;21(3): 431–9.
[97] Lacoste H, Fan TM, de Lorimier LP, et al. Urine N-telopeptide excretion in dogs with appendicular osteosarcoma. J Vet Intern Med 2006;20(2):335–41.
[98] Wypij JM, Fan TM, Fredrickson RL, et al. In vivo and in vitro efficacy of zoledronate for treating oral squamous cell carcinoma in cats. J Vet Intern Med 2008; in press.
[99] Fan TM, de Lorimier LP, Garrett LD, et al. The bone biologic effects of intravenous zoledronate in dogs with malignant osteolysis, submitted for publication.
[100] de Lorimier LP, Fan TM. Bone metabolic effects of single-dose zoledronate in healthy dogs. J Vet Intern Med 2005;19(6):924–7.
[101] Mundy GR. Pathophysiology of cancer-associated hypercalcemia. Semin Oncol 1990;17(2 Suppl 5):10–5.
[102] Mundy GR. Incidence and pathophysiology of hypercalcemia. Calcif Tissue Int 1990;46(Suppl):S3–10.
[103] Rizzoli R, Caverzasio J, Bauss F, et al. Inhibition of bone resorption by the bisphosphonate BM 21.0955 is not associated with an alteration of the renal handling of calcium in rats infused with parathyroid hormone-related protein. Bone 1992;13(4):321–5.
[104] Chisholm MA, Mulloy AL, Taylor AT. Acute management of cancer-related hypercalcemia. Ann Pharmacother 1996;30(5):507–13.
[105] Walls J, Ratcliffe WA, Howell A, et al. Response to IV bisphosphonate therapy in hypercalcaemic patients with and without bone metastases: the role of parathyroid hormone-related protein. Br J Cancer 1994;70(1):169–72.
[106] Hostutler RA, Chew DJ, Jaeger JQ, et al. Uses and effectiveness of pamidronate disodium for treatment of dogs and cats with hypercalcemia. J Vet Intern Med 2005;19(1):29–33.
[107] Kadar E, Rush JE, Wetmore L, et al. Electrolyte disturbances and cardiac arrhythmias in a dog following pamidronate, calcitonin, and furosemide administration for hypercalcemia of malignancy. J Am Anim Hosp Assoc 2004;40(1):75–81.

Anticancer Vaccines

Philip J. Bergman, DVM, MS, PhD[a,b,*]

[a]Brightheart Veterinary Centers, 80 Business Park Drive, Suite 110, Armonk, NY 10504, USA
[b]Memorial Sloan-Kettering Cancer Center, New York, NY, USA

The term *immunity* is derived from the Latin word *immunitas*, which refers to the legal protection afforded to Roman senators holding office. Although the immune system is normally thought of as providing protection against infectious disease, the immune system's ability to recognize and eliminate cancer is the fundamental rationale for the immunotherapy of cancer. Multiple lines of evidence support a role for the immune system in managing cancer, including (1) spontaneous remissions in patients who have cancer and do not have treatment; (2) the presence of tumor-specific cytotoxic T cells within tumor or draining lymph nodes; (3) the presence of monocytic, lymphocytic, and plasmacytic cellular infiltrates in tumors; (4) the increased incidence of some types of cancer in immunosuppressed patients; and (5) documentation of cancer remissions with the use of immunomodulators [1]. With the tools of molecular biology and a greater understanding of mechanisms to harness the immune system, effective tumor immunotherapy is becoming a reality. This new class of therapeutics offers a more targeted, and therefore precise, approach to the treatment of cancer. The recent conditional licensure of a xenogeneic DNA vaccine for advanced canine malignant melanoma (CMM) strongly suggests that immunotherapy can play an extremely important role alongside the classic cancer treatment triad components of surgery, radiation therapy, and chemotherapy; we ardently look forward to immunotherapy playing a larger and larger role in the treatment of cancer in the future.

Any discussion about the potential usefulness of cancer immunotherapeutics predicates a more complete understanding of the principal players in the immune system, which is subsequently briefly reviewed here, before a further discussion on anticancer vaccines and other anticancer immunotherapy strategies.

TUMOR IMMUNOLOGY

The immune system is generally divided into two primary components: the innate immune response and the highly specific but more slowly developing adaptive or acquired immune response. Innate immunity is rapidly acting

*Brightheart Veterinary Centers, 80 Business Park Drive, Suite 110, Armonk, NY 10504.
E-mail address: pbergman@brightheartvet.com

but typically not extremely specific and includes physicochemical barriers (eg, skin, mucosa); blood proteins, such as complement; phagocytic cells (macrophages, neutrophils, dendritic cells [DCs], and natural killer [NK] cells); and cytokines, which coordinate and regulate the cells involved in innate immunity. Adaptive immunity is thought of as the acquired arm of immunity that allows for exquisite specificity, an ability to remember the previous existence of the pathogen and to differentiate self from nonself, and, importantly, the ability to respond more vigorously on repeat exposure to the pathogen. Adaptive immunity consists of T and B lymphocytes. The T cells are further divided by cluster of differentiation (CD) and major histocompatibility complex (MHC) class into T helper cells (CD4 positive and MHC II), and T cytotoxic cells (CD8 positive and MHC I). B lymphocytes produce antibodies (humoral system) that may activate complement, enhance phagocytosis of opsonized target cells, and induce antibody-dependent cellular cytotoxicity (ADCC). B-cell responses to tumors are thought by many investigators to be less important than the development of T-cell–mediated immunity, but there is little evidence to support this notion fully [2]. The innate and adaptive arms of immunity are not mutually exclusive; they are linked by (1) the innate response's ability to stimulate and influence the nature of the adaptive response and (2) the sharing of effector mechanisms between innate and adaptive immune responses.

Immune responses can be further separated by whether they are induced by exposure to a foreign antigen (an "active" response) or if they are transferred through serum or lymphocytes from an immunized individual (a "passive" response). Although both approaches have the ability to be extremely specific for an antigen of interest, one important difference is the inability of passive approaches to confer memory. The principal components of the active/adaptive immune system are lymphocytes, antigen-presenting cells, and effector cells. Furthermore, responses can be subdivided by whether they are specific for a certain antigen or a nonspecific response whereby immunity is attempted to be conferred by upregulating the immune system without a specific target. These definitions are helpful because they allow methodologies to be more completely characterized, such as active specific and passive nonspecific, for example.

The idea that the immune system may actively prevent the development of neoplasia is termed *cancer immunosurveillance*. Sound scientific evidence supports some aspects of this hypothesis [3,4], including the following: (1) interferon (IFN)-γ protects mice against the growth of tumors; (2) mice lacking IFNγ receptor were more sensitive to chemically induced sarcomas than normal mice and were more likely to develop tumors spontaneously; (3) mice lacking major components of the adaptive immune response (T and B cells) have a high rate of spontaneous tumors; and (4) mice that lack IFNγ and B/T cells develop tumors, especially at a young age.

There are significant barriers to the generation of effective antitumor immunity by the host. Many tumors evade surveillance mechanisms and grow in immunocompetent hosts, as easily illustrated by the overwhelming numbers of people and animals succumbing to cancer. There are multiple ways in which tumors evade the immune response, including the following: (1) immunosuppressive cytokine production (eg, transforming growth factor [TGF]-β, interleukin [IL]-10) [5,6]; (2) impaired DC function by means of inactivation ("anergy") or poor DC maturation through changes in IL-6/IL-10/vascular endothelial growth factor (VEGF)/granulocyte macrophage colony-stimulating factor (GM-CSF) [7]; (3) induction of cells called regulatory T cells (Treg), which were initially called suppressor T cells (CD4/CD25/CTLA-4/GITR/Foxp3-positive cells, which can suppress tumor-specific CD4/CD8+ T cells) [8,9]; (4) MHC I loss through structural defects, changes in B2-microglobulin synthesis, defects in transporter-associated antigen processing, or actual MHC I gene loss (ie, allelic, locus loss); and (5) MHC I antigen presentation loss through B7-1 attenuation (B7-1 is an important costimulatory molecule for CD28-mediated T-cell receptor and MHC engagement) when the MHC system in MHC I loss remains intact.

NONSPECIFIC TUMOR IMMUNOTHERAPY

Dr. William Coley, a New York surgeon in the early 1900s, noted that some patients who had cancer and developed incidental bacterial infections survived longer than those without infection [10]. Coley developed a bacterial "vaccine" (killed cultures of *Serratia marcescens* and *Streptococcus pyogenes* ["Coley's toxins"]) to treat people with sarcomas, which provided complete response rates of approximately 15%. Unfortunately, high failure rates and significant side effects led to discontinuation of this approach. His seminal work laid the foundation for nonspecific modulation of the immune response in the treatment of cancer. Nonspecific tumor immunotherapy approaches are numerous, and relevant examples are listed in Table 1 [11–34].

CANCER VACCINES

The ultimate goal for a cancer vaccine is elicitation of an antitumor immune response that results in clinical regression of a tumor or its metastases. Responses to cancer vaccines may take several months or more to appear because of the slower speed of induction of the adaptive arm of the immune system, as outlined in Table 2.

There are numerous types of tumor vaccines in phase I through III human trials across a wide range of tumor types. The immune system detects tumors through specific tumor-associated antigens (TAAs) that are recognized by cytotoxic T lymphocytes (CTLs) and antibodies. TAAs may be common to a particular tumor type; may be unique to an individual tumor; or may arise from mutated gene products, such as ras, p53, p21, or others. Although unique TAAs may be more immunogenic than the other aforementioned shared tumor antigens, they are not practical targets because of their narrow specificity. Most shared tumor antigens are normal cellular antigens that are overexpressed in tumors. The first group to be identified was termed *cancer testes antigens* because of expression in normal testes, but they are also found in

Table 1
Examples of nonspecific immunotherapy approaches

Immunotherapy approach	Agent(s)	Tumor types investigated with this approach in veterinary medicine	Reference
Biologic response modifiers	Bacille Calmette-Guérin (BCG)	Mammary and bladder carcinoma	[11–14]
	Corynebacterium parvum	Mammary carcinoma and melanoma	[11,15]
	Mycobacterial cell wall–DNA complexes (MCCs)	Bladder carcinoma and osteosarcoma	VCS abstracts
	Attenuated Salmonella (VNP20009)	Various tumors	[16]
	Bacterial superantigens	Various tumors, including melanoma	[17]
	Oncolytic viruses (Newcastle disease virus, reovirus, vesicular stomatitis virus, vaccinia, adenovirus, herpes simplex virus, canine distemper virus)	Various tumors, including lymphoma	[18–21]
	Liposome-encapsulated muramyl tripeptide-phosphatidylethanolamine (L-MTP-PE)	Hemangiosarcoma, melanoma, and osteosarcoma	[22–24]
	Recombinant canine granulocyte macrophage colony-stimulating factor (rcGM-CSF)	Melanoma	[22,25,37]
	Imiquimod (Aldara)	Bowen's-like disease (multicentric intraepithelial squamous cell carcinoma)	VCS abstract
	Liposome-DNA complexes	Osteosarcoma	[26]
Recombinant cytokines	IL-2	Feline fibrosarcoma and canine melanoma	[38,42]
	Liposomal IL-2	Osteosarcoma	[27]
	IL-12	Hemangiosarcoma, feline soft tissue sarcoma, and in vitro immunostimulation	[28–30]
	IL-18	In vitro	[31]
	IFNs	In vitro	[32–34]

Abbreviation: VCS, Veterinary Cancer Society.

Table 2
Comparison of chemotherapy and antitumor vaccines

Treatment type	Mechanism of action	Specificity	Sensitivity	Response time	Durability of response
Chemotherapy	Cytotoxicity	Poor	Variable	Hours to days	Variable
Antitumor vaccine	Immune response	Good	Good	Weeks to months	Variable to long

melanoma and various other solid tumors, such as the MAGE/BAGE gene family. This article highlights those tumor vaccine approaches that seem to hold particular promise in human clinical trials and some that have been tested to date in veterinary medicine.

A variety of approaches have been taken to focus the immune system on the aforementioned targets, including (1) whole cell or tumor cell lysate vaccines (autologous, or made from a patient's own tumor tissue; allogeneic, or made from individuals within a species bearing the same type of cancer; or whole cell vaccines from γ-irradiated tumor cell lines with or without immunostimulatory cytokines) [35–38]; (2) DNA vaccines that immunize with syngeneic or xenogeneic (different species than the recipient) plasmid DNA designed to elicit antigen-specific humoral and cellular immunity (to be discussed in more detail elsewhere in this article); (3) viral vector-based or other methodologies designed to deliver genes encoding TAAs or immunostimulatory cytokines [39,40]; (4) DC vaccines that are commonly loaded or transfected with TAAs, DNA or RNA from TAAs, or tumor lysates [41]; (5) adoptive cell transfer (the "transfer" of specific populations of immune effector cells to generate a more powerful and focused antitumor immune response); (6) cytokine approaches [42]; and (7) antibody approaches, such as monoclonal antibodies [43], anti-idiotype antibodies (an idiotype is an immunoglobulin sequence unique to each B lymphocyte; therefore, antibodies directed against these idiotypes are referred to as anti-idiotype), or conjugated antibodies. The ideal cancer immunotherapy agent would be able to discriminate between cancer and normal cells (ie, specificity), be potent enough to kill small or large numbers of tumor cells (ie, sensitivity) and, finally, be able to prevent recurrence of the tumor (ie, durability).

This author has developed a xenogeneic DNA vaccine program for melanoma at the Animal Medical Center in collaboration with human investigators from Memorial Sloan-Kettering Cancer Center and industrial partner Merial [44,45]. Preclinical and clinical studies by this author's laboratory and others have shown that xenogeneic DNA vaccination with tyrosinase family members (eg, tyrosinase, GP100, GP75, others) can produce immune responses resulting in tumor rejection or protection and prolongation of survival, whereas syngeneic vaccination with orthologous DNA does not induce immune responses [46]. These studies provided the impetus for development of a xenogeneic

DNA vaccine program in CMM. Cohorts of dogs received increasing doses of xenogeneic plasmid DNA encoding human tyrosinase (huTyr), murine GP75 (muGP75), murine tyrosinase (muTyr), muTyr with or without human GM-CSF (both administered as plasmid DNA), or muTyr "off study" administered intramuscularly biweekly for a total of four vaccinations. Minimal to mild pain was noted on vaccination, and one dog experienced vitiligo. The authors and his colleagues have recently investigated antibody responses in dogs vaccinated with HuTyr and found two- to fivefold increases in circulating antibodies to huTyr, which can cross react to canine tyrosinase, suggesting the breaking of tolerance [47]. The clinical results with prolongation in survival have been reported previously [44,45]. The results of these trials demonstrate that xenogeneic DNA vaccination in CMM (1) is safe, (2) leads to the development of antityrosinase antibodies, (3) is potentially therapeutic, and (4) is an attractive candidate for further evaluation in an adjuvant minimal residual disease phase II setting for CMM. A US Department of Agriculture (USDA) licensure study of huTyr in dogs with advanced malignant melanoma was initiated in April 2006, which led to USDA conditional licensure in March 2007. This is the first approved vaccine for the treatment of cancer across species in the United States. The xenogeneic DNA vaccine platform represents an interesting mechanism for exploration of immune responses and anticancer responses for other malignancies. To this end, the author and his colleagues have recently initiated a phase I trial of murine CD20 for dogs and cats with B-cell lymphoma [48].

Tumor immunology and immunotherapy is one of the most exciting and rapidly expanding fields at present. Significant resources are focused on mechanisms to stimulate an antitumor immune response maximally while minimizing the immunosuppressive aspects of the tumor microenvironment simultaneously. The recent elucidation and blockade of immunosuppressive cytokines (eg, TGFβ, IL-10, IL-13) or the negative costimulatory molecule CTLA-4 [49] may dramatically improve cell-mediated immunity to tumors. Immunotherapy is unlikely to become a sole modality in the treatment of cancer; the traditional modalities of surgery, radiation, and chemotherapy are extremely likely to be used in combination with immunotherapy in the future. Like any form of anticancer treatment, immunotherapy seems to work best in a minimal residual disease setting, suggesting that its most appropriate use is likely to be in an adjuvant setting with local tumor therapies, such as surgery or radiation. Similarly, the long held belief that chemotherapy attenuates immune responses from cancer vaccines is beginning to be disproved through investigations on a variety of levels [50,51]. In fact, mechanisms to induce cancer cell lysis through chemotherapy or other means after anticancer vaccination may induce increased cancer antigen presentation to an already primed immune system, thereby leading to a boosting of the immune response.

In summary, the future looks extremely bright for immunotherapy. Similarly, the veterinary oncology profession is uniquely able to contribute greatly to the many advances to come in this field. Unfortunately, what works in a mouse often does not reflect the outcome in human patients who have cancer. Therefore, comparative immunotherapy studies using veterinary patients may be better able to "bridge" murine and human studies. To this end, a large number of cancers in dogs and cats seem to be remarkably stronger models for counterpart human tumors than presently available murine model systems. This is likely attributable to a variety of reasons, including but not limited to extreme similarities in the biology of the tumors (eg, chemoresistance, radioresistance, sharing metastatic phenotypes, site selectivity), spontaneous syngeneic cancer (typically versus an induced or xenogeneic cancer in murine models), and, finally, the fact that the dogs and cats spontaneously developing these tumors are outbred and immune competent and live in the same environment as human beings. The field of veterinary tumor immunotherapy is greatly indebted to the tireless work and seeds laid by MacEwen [52]. This author ardently looks forward to the time when immunotherapy plays a significant role in the treatment or prevention of cancer in human and veterinary patients.

References

[1] Bergman PJ. Biologic response modification. In: Rosenthal RC, editor. Veterinary oncology secrets. 1st edition. Philadelphia: Hanley & Belfus, Inc.; 2001. p. 79–82.
[2] Reilly RT, Emens LA, Jaffee EM. Humoral and cellular immune responses: independent forces or collaborators in the fight against cancer? Curr Opin Investig Drugs 2001;2(1):133–5.
[3] Smyth MJ, Godfrey DI, Trapani JA. A fresh look at tumor immunosurveillance and immunotherapy. Nat Immunol 2001;2(4):293–9.
[4] Wallace ME, Smyth MJ. The role of natural killer cells in tumor control—effectors and regulators of adaptive immunity. Springer Semin Immunopathol 2005;27(1):49–64.
[5] Catchpole B, Gould SM, Kellett-Gregory LM, et al. Immunosuppressive cytokines in the regional lymph node of a dog suffering from oral malignant melanoma. J Small Anim Pract 2002;43(10):464–7.
[6] Zagury D, Gallo RC. Anti-cytokine Ab immune therapy: present status and perspectives. Drug Discov Today 2004;9(2):72–81.
[7] Morse MA, Mosca PJ, Clay TM, et al. Dendritic cell maturation in active immunotherapy strategies. Expert Opin Biol Ther 2002;2(1):35–43.
[8] Yamaguchi T, Sakaguchi S. Regulatory T cells in immune surveillance and treatment of cancer. Semin Cancer Biol 2006;16(2):115–23.
[9] Biller BJ, Elmslie RE, Burnett RC, et al. Use of FoxP3 expression to identify regulatory T cells in healthy dogs and dogs with cancer. Vet Immunol Immunopathol 2007;116(1–2):69–78.
[10] Richardson MA, Ramirez T, Russell NC, et al. Coley toxins immunotherapy: a retrospective review. Altern Ther Health Med 1999;5(3):42–7.
[11] Parodi AL, Misdorp W, Mialot JP, et al. Intratumoral BCG and Corynebacterium parvum therapy of canine mammary tumours before radical mastectomy. Cancer Immunol Immunother 1983;15(3):172–7.
[12] Bostock DE, Gorman NT. Intravenous BCG therapy of mammary carcinoma in bitches after surgical excision of the primary tumour. Eur J Cancer 1978;14(8):879–83.
[13] vd Meijden AP, Steerenberg PA, de Jong WH, et al. The effects of intravesical and intradermal application of a new B.C.G. on the dog bladder. Urol Res 1986;14(4):207–10.
[14] MacEwen EG. Approaches to cancer therapy using biological response modifiers. Vet Clin North Am Small Anim Pract 1985;15(3):667–88.
[15] MacEwen EG, Patnaik AK, Harvey HJ, et al. Canine oral melanoma: comparison of surgery versus surgery plus Corynebacterium parvum. Cancer Invest 1986;4(5):397–402.

[16] Thamm DH, Kurzman ID, King I, et al. Systemic administration of an attenuated, tumor-targeting Salmonella typhimurium to dogs with spontaneous neoplasia: phase I evaluation. Clin Cancer Res 2005;11(13):4827–34.
[17] Dow SW, Elmslie RE, Willson AP, et al. In vivo tumor transfection with superantigen plus cytokine genes induces tumor regression and prolongs survival in dogs with malignant melanoma. J Clin Invest 1998;101(11):2406–14.
[18] Suter SE, Chein MB, von M, et al. In vitro canine distemper virus infection of canine lymphoid cells: a prelude to oncolytic therapy for lymphoma. Clin Cancer Res 2005;11(4):1579–87.
[19] Le LP, Rivera AA, Glasgow JN, et al. Infectivity enhancement for adenoviral transduction of canine osteosarcoma cells. Gene Ther 2006;13(5):389–99.
[20] Hemminki A, Kanerva A, Kremer EJ, et al. A canine conditionally replicating adenovirus for evaluating oncolytic virotherapy in a syngeneic animal model. Mol Ther 2003;7(2):163–73.
[21] Hodes ME, Morgan S, Hubbard JD, et al. Tissue culture and animal studies with an oncolytic bovine enterovirus (bovine enterovirus 1). Cancer Res 1973;33(10):2408–14.
[22] MacEwen EG, Kurzman ID, Vail DM, et al. Adjuvant therapy for melanoma in dogs: results of randomized clinical trials using surgery, liposome-encapsulated muramyl tripeptide, and granulocyte macrophage colony-stimulating factor. Clin Cancer Res 1999;5(12):4249–58.
[23] Kurzman ID, MacEwen EG, Rosenthal RC, et al. Adjuvant therapy for osteosarcoma in dogs: results of randomized clinical trials using combined liposome-encapsulated muramyl tripeptide and cisplatin. Clin Cancer Res 1995;1(12):1595–601.
[24] Vail DM, MacEwen EG, Kurzman ID, et al. Liposome-encapsulated muramyl tripeptide phosphatidylethanolamine adjuvant immunotherapy for splenic hemangiosarcoma in the dog: a randomized multi-institutional clinical trial. Clin Cancer Res 1995;1(10):1165–70.
[25] Hogge GS, Burkholder JK, Culp J, et al. Development of human granulocyte-macrophage colony-stimulating factor-transfected tumor cell vaccines for the treatment of spontaneous canine cancer. Hum Gene Ther 1998;9(13):1851–61.
[26] Dow S, Elmslie R, Kurzman I, et al. Phase I study of liposome-DNA complexes encoding the interleukin-2 gene in dogs with osteosarcoma lung metastases. Hum Gene Ther 2005;16(8):937–46.
[27] Khanna C, Anderson PM, Hasz DE, et al. Interleukin-2 liposome inhalation therapy is safe and effective for dogs with spontaneous pulmonary metastases. Cancer 1997;79(7):1409–21.
[28] Akhtar N, Padilla ML, Dickerson EB, et al. Interleukin-12 inhibits tumor growth in a novel angiogenesis canine hemangiosarcoma xenograft model. Neoplasia 2004;6(2):106–16.
[29] Phillips BS, Padilla ML, Dickerson EB, et al. Immunostimulatory effects of human recombinant interleukin-12 on peripheral blood mononuclear cells from normal dogs. Vet Immunol Immunopathol 1999;70(3–4):189–201.
[30] Siddiqui F, Li CY, Larue SM, et al. A phase I trial of hyperthermia-induced interleukin-12 gene therapy in spontaneously arising feline soft tissue sarcomas. Mol Cancer Ther 2007;6(1):380–9.
[31] Okano F, Yamada K. Canine interleukin-18 induces apoptosis and enhances Fas ligand mRNA expression in a canine carcinoma cell line. Anticancer Res 2000;20(5B):3411–5.
[32] Kruth SA. Biological response modifiers: interferons, interleukins, recombinant products, liposomal products. Vet Clin North Am Small Anim Pract 1998;28(2):269–95.
[33] Tateyama S, Priosoeryanto BP, Yamaguchi R, et al. In vitro growth inhibition activities of recombinant feline interferon on all lines derived from canine tumours. Res Vet Sci 1995;59(3):275–7.
[34] Whitley EM, Bird AC, Zucker KE, et al. Modulation by canine interferon-gamma of major histocompatibility complex and tumor-associated antigen expression in canine mammary tumor and melanoma cell lines. Anticancer Res 1995;15(3):923–9.

[35] Alexander AN, Huelsmeyer MK, Mitzey A, et al. Development of an allogeneic whole-cell tumor vaccine expressing xenogeneic gp100 and its implementation in a phase II clinical trial in canine patients with malignant melanoma. Cancer Immunol Immunother 2006;55(4):433–42.
[36] U'Ren LW, Biller BJ, Elmslie RE, et al. Evaluation of a novel tumor vaccine in dogs with hemangiosarcoma. J Vet Intern Med 2007;21(1):113–20.
[37] Hogge GS, Burkholder JK, Culp J, et al. Preclinical development of human granulocyte-macrophage colony-stimulating factor-transfected melanoma cell vaccine using established canine cell lines and normal dogs. Cancer Gene Ther 1999;6(1):26–36.
[38] Quintin-Colonna F, Devauchelle P, Fradelizi D, et al. Gene therapy of spontaneous canine melanoma and feline fibrosarcoma by intratumoral administration of histoincompatible cells expressing human interleukin-2. Gene Ther 1996;3(12):1104–12.
[39] Jourdier TM, Moste C, Bonnet MC, et al. Local immunotherapy of spontaneous feline fibrosarcomas using recombinant poxviruses expressing interleukin 2 (IL2). Gene Ther 2003;10(26):2126–32.
[40] Milner RJ, Salute M, Crawford C, et al. The immune response to disialoganglioside GD3 vaccination in normal dogs: a melanoma surface antigen vaccine. Vet Immunol Immunopathol 2006;114(3–4):273–84.
[41] Gyorffy S, Rodriguez-Lecompte JC, Woods JP, et al. Bone marrow-derived dendritic cell vaccination of dogs with naturally occurring melanoma by using human gp100 antigen. J Vet Intern Med 2005;19(1):56–63.
[42] Helfand SC, Soergel SA, Donner RL, et al. Potential to involve multiple effector cells with human recombinant interleukin-2 and antiganglioside monoclonal antibodies in a canine malignant melanoma immunotherapy model. J Immunother Emphasis Tumor Immunol 1994;16(3):188–97.
[43] Jeglum KA. Chemoimmunotherapy of canine lymphoma with adjuvant canine monoclonal antibody 231. Vet Clin North Am Small Anim Pract 1996;26(1):73–85.
[44] Bergman PJ, Camps-Palau MA, McKnight JA, et al. Development of a xenogeneic DNA vaccine program for canine malignant melanoma at the Animal Medical Center. Vaccine 2006;24(21):4582–5.
[45] Bergman PJ, McKnight J, Novosad A, et al. Long-term survival of dogs with advanced malignant melanoma after DNA vaccination with xenogeneic human tyrosinase: a phase I trial. Clin Cancer Res 2003;9(4):1284–90.
[46] Srinivasan R, Wolchok JD. Tumor antigens for cancer immunotherapy: therapeutic potential of xenogeneic DNA vaccines. J Transl Med 2004;2(1):12–24.
[47] Liao JC, Gregor P, Wolchok JD, et al. Vaccination with human tyrosinase DNA induces antibody responses in dogs with advanced melanoma. Cancer Immun 2006;6:8–18.
[48] Palomba ML, Roberts WK, Dao T, et al. CD8+ T-cell-dependent immunity following xenogeneic DNA immunization against CD20 in a tumor challenge model of B-cell lymphoma. Clin Cancer Res 2005;11(1):370–9.
[49] Peggs KS, Quezada SA, Korman AJ, et al. Principles and use of anti-CTLA4 antibody in human cancer immunotherapy. Curr Opin Immunol 2006;18(2):206–13.
[50] Walter CU, Biller BJ, Lana SE, et al. Effects of chemotherapy on immune responses in dogs with cancer. J Vet Intern Med 2006;20(2):342–7.
[51] Emens LA, Jaffee EM. Leveraging the activity of tumor vaccines with cytotoxic chemotherapy. Cancer Res 2005;65(18):8059–64.
[52] MacEwen EG. An immunologic approach to the treatment of cancer. Vet Clin North Am 1977;7(1):65–75.

The Role of Small Molecule Inhibitors for Veterinary Patients

Cheryl A. London, DVM, PhD

Department of Veterinary Biosciences, College of Veterinary Medicine, The Ohio State University, 454 VMAB, 1925 Coffey Road, Columbus, OH 43210, USA

Advances in molecular techniques have provided important new insights into the biology of cancer. Perhaps most relevant for the development of new treatments has been the finding that cellular components regulating signal transduction, cell survival, and cell proliferation are dysregulated in neoplastic cells. In many instances, cancer cells depend on these dysregulated pathways; as such, they have arisen as promising targets for therapeutic intervention. A variety of small molecule inhibitors that target specific cellular proteins have now been approved for the treatment of human cancer, and many more are likely to become available in the near future. In many instances, these inhibitors have exhibited significant clinical efficacy and their biologic activity is likely to be further enhanced as combination regimens with standard treatment modalities are explored. This article reviews the current status of small molecule inhibitors in human oncology and discusses their application to veterinary patients that have cancer.

KINASE INHIBITORS: THE HUMAN EXPERIENCE

Protein kinases are critical players in normal cell signal transduction, acting to regulate cell growth and differentiation tightly. Kinases work through the act of phosphorylation; they bind ATP and use this to add phosphate groups to key residues on themselves (termed *autophosphorylation*) and on other molecules, resulting in a downstream signal inside the cell. In most cases, kinase phosphorylation is initiated by an external signal, such as growth factor binding. The resultant signaling cascade induces sequential phosphorylation and activation of cytoplasmic kinases, ultimately leading to alterations in gene transcription that have an impact on cell proliferation and survival (reviewed by London [1]). This process is usually in response to external signals generated from growth factors or other stimuli that initiate the cascade. Protein kinases may be located at the cell surface, in the cytoplasm, or in the nucleus, and they are typically divided into three categories: tyrosine kinases that are phosphorylated on tyrosine,

E-mail address: london.20@osu.edu

serine-threonine kinases that phosphorylated on serine and threonine, and mixed kinases that are phosphorylated on all three amino acids.

Those tyrosine kinases expressed on the cell surface that bind growth factors are termed *receptor tyrosine kinases* (RTKs); 58 of the 90 known tyrosine kinases are RTKs. These RTKs are composed of an extracellular ligand binding domain, a transmembrane domain, and a cytoplasmic tyrosine kinase domain that serves to regulate phosphorylation events positively and negatively [2,3]. The RTKs usually exist as monomers, and dimerization is induced through growth factor binding, which results in autophosphorylation and subsequent downstream signaling. Examples of RTKs include Kit, Met, Axl, and epidermal growth factor receptor (EGFR), all of which have recently been shown to play prominent roles in particular forms of cancer [4–7].

In addition to regulating normal cell function, certain RTKs play a critical role in the process of tumor angiogenesis. These include vascular endothelial growth factor (VEGF) receptor (VEGFR), platelet-derived growth factor (PDGF) receptor (PDGFR), fibroblast growth factor (FGF) receptor (FGFR), and Tie1/2 [8–11]. VEGFRs are expressed on vascular endothelium, and VEGF-VEGFR interactions are critical for endothelial migration and proliferation [8]. PDGF and PDGFR are expressed in stroma and pericytes, and PDGF can induce promote angiogenesis in some studies [10,11]. FGF is synergistic with VEGF to induce the expression of VEGF [10]. Finally, Tie1 and Tie2 are involved in the recruitment of pericytes and smooth muscle cells and in maintaining vascular integrity [12].

With respect to the cytoplasmic kinases, two major pathways have been the focus of significant research regarding tumorigenesis (Fig. 1). The first of these involves members of the RAS-RAF-MEK-ERK/p38/JNK families [13,14]. These are serine-threonine kinases that modulate cell cycling and apoptosis by means of translocation of ERK/p38/JNK into the nucleus after phosphorylation. Dysregulation of this pathway has been identified in human cancers, with RAS mutations known to be present in lung, colon, and various hematologic malignancies [14]. Recently, B-Raf mutations have been identified in cutaneous human melanomas, suggesting a critical role for this kinase in melanoma development [15–17].

The second major cytoplasmic pathway involves phosphatidyl inositol 3 kinase (PI3K) and includes the downstream signal transducers Akt, nuclear factor-κB (NF-κB), and mTOR, among others [18,19]. Akt modulates the function of several substrates involved in the regulation of cell survival and cycling, such as BAD, mTOR, p21, and p27, acting to inhibit apoptosis and stimulate cell cycling and growth [18–20]. PI3K and Akt are overexpressed in several cancers through gene amplification, including those of the cervix, ovary, pancreas, and breast [21–24]. The PI3K pathway is also inappropriately activated through loss of a regulatory protein PTEN (a phosphatase), which inhibits Akt through dephosphorylation [18,25,26]. PTEN mutations are found in a variety of human cancers and result in permanent PI3K signaling and uncontrolled growth [25].

Dysfunction of protein kinases has been extensively characterized in human malignancies and is just beginning to be investigated in canine and feline tumors. They may be dysregulated by mutation, overexpression, the generation of fusion proteins from chromosomal translocation, or autocrine loops of activation through coexpression of growth factor and receptor [27]. The net consequence of this dysregulation is persistent cell signaling in the absence of appropriate negative regulation, thereby stimulating uncontrolled cell growth and survival. In most instances, a particular type of cancer exhibits dysregulation of a specific kinase (often referred to as "oncogene addiction"), permitting the development of therapies that target that kinase or its downstream signaling elements.

Although several strategies exist for targeting protein kinases, the most successful approach to date has been the use of small molecule inhibitors. These typically work by blocking the ATP binding site of kinases, essentially acting as competitive inhibitors [28–30]. In the absence of ATP binding, the kinase is not able to phosphorylate itself or initiate downstream signaling. To develop inhibitors specific for particular proteins, the ATP binding pockets of many kinases have been characterized to permit the rational design of competitive inhibitors that exhibit activity against a restricted set of kinases, thereby limiting off-target effects (ie, inhibition of other nontarget kinases). Such inhibitors are often easy to synthesize in large quantities, are frequently orally bioavailable, and can readily enter cells to gain access to the intended target. Some examples of kinases known to be dysregulated in human cancers are discussed in this article, along with the targeted therapeutics used to inhibit them.

Perhaps the most successful small molecule kinase inhibitor developed to date is Gleevec (STI571, imatinib mesylate; Novartis, East Hanover, New Jersey), an orally administered drug that blocks the activity of a cytoplasmic kinase called Abl. This drug was designed specifically to target the constitutively active Bcr-Abl fusion protein found in approximately 90% of human patients who have chronic myelogenous leukemia (CML) [31,32]. Numerous clinical trials of Gleevec have been completed in patients who have CML with exciting results [33–38]. For those individuals in the chronic phase of the disease, Gleevec induces a remission rate close to 95% and most patients remain in remission for longer than 1 year. Unfortunately, remission rates are much lower for patients in blast crisis (20%–50%), lasting, on average, less than 10 months. Resistance to Gleevec is often attributable to Bcr-Abl gene amplification and mutations in the ATP binding pocket that prevent appropriate binding of the inhibitor [39,40].

During screening for off-target effects, Gleevec was found to block the ATP binding site of another kinase, Kit, an RTK normally expressed on hematopoietic stem cells, on melanocytes, in the central nervous system, and on mast cells [41]. Dysregulation of Kit has been identified in several human cancers, including systemic mastocytosis [42], acute myelogenous leukemia (AML) [43], and gastrointestinal stromal tumors (GISTs) [44,45]. Interestingly, 60% to 90% of the GISTs possess mutations in the juxtamembrane domain of Kit, resulting in constitutive activation in the absence of growth factor stimulation [46,47].

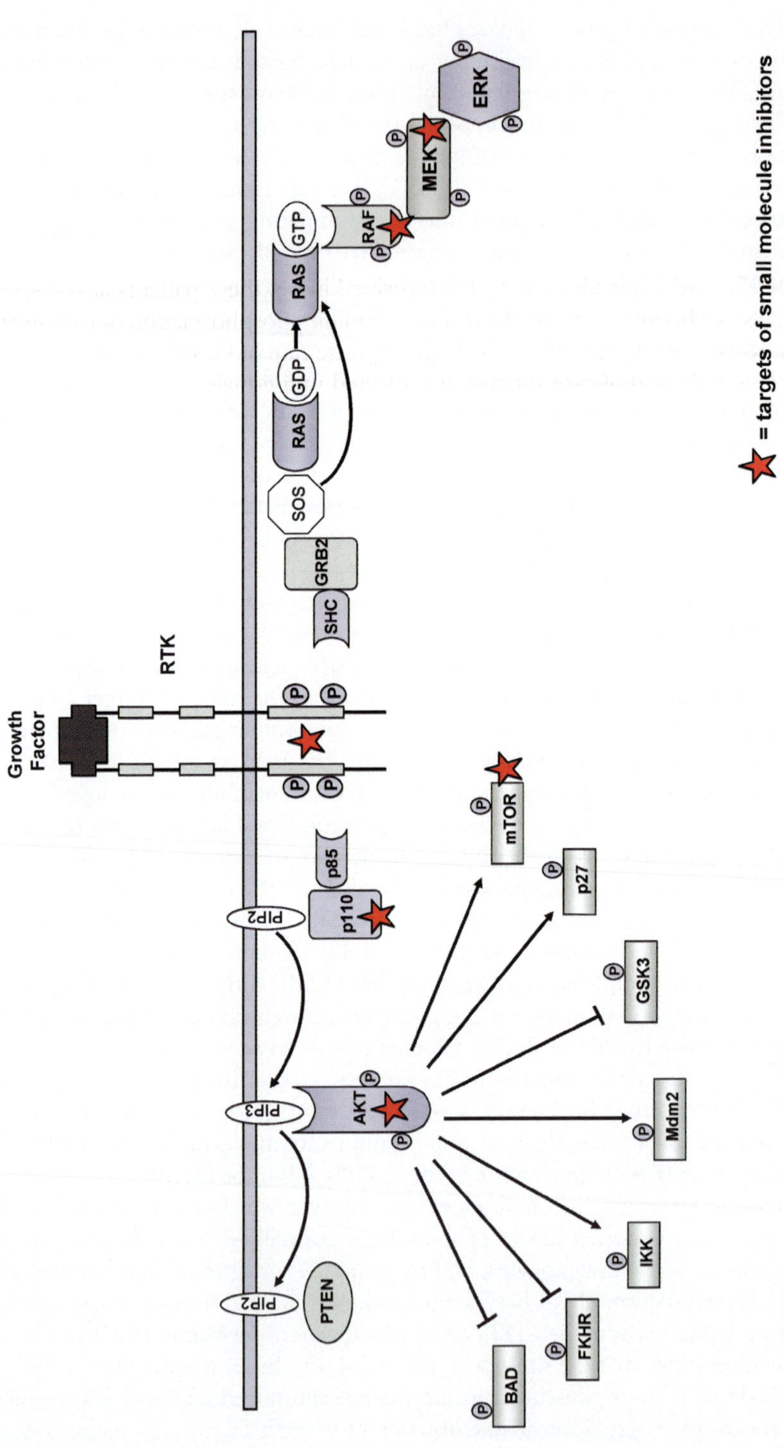
Growth Factor
RTK
SHC
GRB2
SOS
RAS
GDP
RAS
GTP
RAF
MEK
ERK
P
PIP2
PIP3
PIP2
p85
p110
PTEN
AKT
mTOR
p27
GSK3
Mdm2
IKK
FKHR
BAD
= targets of small molecule inhibitors

GISTs are known to be resistant to chemotherapy, and the prognosis for affected individuals is usually poor [48,49]. Given the high prevalence of Kit dysregulation in this tumor type, it was reasonable to assume that inhibition of Kit signaling would induce responses in affected patients. As predicted, clinical trials of Gleevec in the treatment of GISTs induced responses in 50% to 70% of patients, which is far better than the 5% response rate to standard chemotherapy. Additionally, a small number of patients who have GISTs have tumors that do not possess Kit mutations but instead have activating mutations in PDGFRα, which is also a receptor tyrosine kinase; these patients also respond to Gleevec because the drug is known to inhibit phosphorylation of this protein kinase as well [50]. Based on the high response rate of GISTs to Gleevec, it has become standard-of-care therapy for affected individuals.

The small molecule inhibitor SUTENT (SU11248, sunitinib; Pfizer, New York, New York) was developed to block the activity of the split kinase family, including VEGFR, PDGFR, and Kit [51]. Like Gleevec, SUTENT sits in the ATP binding pocket of these receptors. Clinical activity of SUTENT was demonstrated in patients who had neuroendocrine, colon, and breast cancers in phase I and II studies. Definitive efficacy was further demonstrated in patients who had Gleevec-resistant GISTs (61% demonstrated disease regression or stable disease lasting longer than 4 months) and renal cell carcinoma who had failed interleukin (IL)-2 or interferon therapy (40% achieved a partial response, whereas an additional 25% experienced stable disease) [51].

Another orally active small molecule inhibitor that has been successful in treating human cancers is gefitinib (Iressa; Astra Zeneca, Wilmington, Delaware). This drug inhibits signaling by EGFR (a receptor tyrosine kinase); like Gleevec, it acts as a competitive inhibitor of ATP binding [52,53]. The EGFR family is an attractive target for inhibition, because many human cancers, including breast, lung cancer, and bladder carcinomas, overexpress one or more family members [5]. In human patients, Iressa has demonstrated clinical activity in non–small-cell lung cancer (NSCLC), with 12% to 20% of patients experiencing complete or partial responses and an additional 30% to

Fig. 1. Cytoplasmic signal transduction. Ras pathway: activated receptor tyrosine kinases recruits SOS to the plasma membrane through binding of SHC and GRB2. SOS replaces bound guanosine diphosphate (GDP) with guanosine triphosphate (GTP), thereby activating RAS. The downstream target RAF is then phosphorylated by RAS, leading to subsequent activation of MEK and then ERK. ERK has several substrates in the nucleus and in the cytoplasm that regulate cell cycle progression. Current targets of therapeutic intervention are indicated. PI3K pathways: after receptor tyrosine kinase activation, PI3 kinase is recruited to the phosphorylated receptor through binding of the p85 adaptor subunit, leading to activation of the catalytic subunit (p110). This activation results in the generation of the second-messenger phosphatidylinositol-3,4,5-triphosphate (PIP3). PIP3 recruits AKT to the membrane; after its phosphorylation, several downstream targets are subsequently phosphorylated leading to their activation or inhibition. The cumulative effect results in cell survival, growth, and proliferation. Current targets of therapeutic intervention are indicated.

40% of patients experiencing stable disease [5,52]. The likelihood of response to Iressa and other EGFR inhibitors is now known to depend on the presence of a point mutation in EGFR that induces prolonged signal transduction after stimulation by its ligand epidermal growth factor (EGF). This results in an increased duration of downstream signal transduction, promoting uncontrolled growth and survival. Interestingly, this mutation is primarily found in patients who have never smoked but have developed a particular histopathologic subset of lung cancer, bronchoalveolar carcinoma [54]. Unfortunately, Iressa has demonstrated little activity against breast cancer, but promising results have been observed for head and neck, prostatic, and ovarian cancers when it is used as a single agent [5,52,53].

B-Raf is a cytoplasmic serine-threonine kinase that connects Ras signals with the mitogen activated protein (MAP) kinase pathway. It is now known that approximately 60% of human cutaneous melanomas possess a mutation in B-Raf (V599E) that induces a conformational change in the protein mimicking its activated form, thus resulting in constitutive downstream MAP kinase signaling [55,56]. Given the high frequency of B-Raf mutations in human melanomas and the lack of effective systemic treatment strategies, a variety of approaches to inhibit this pathway have been developed. Sorafenib (BAY 43-9006; Bayer, Morristown, New Jersey) is derived from the bis-aryl ureas and was initially identified through screening of thousands of medicinal chemistry compounds for activity against RAF [57–59]. Studies are currently underway to evaluate the potential efficacy of this drug in malignant cutaneous melanoma. Like other small molecule inhibitors, Sorafenib exhibits off-target effects, including VEGFR, Kit, and PDGFR, and, as such, has demonstrated clinical activity in the treatment of several other cancers (eg, renal cell carcinoma, sarcomas) in phase II and III clinical trials [60].

Several other small molecule protein kinase inhibitors are currently under development or entering clinical trials at this time. These include inhibitors of the MAP kinase pathway, Src, STAT3, Akt, PI3K, and Met, all of which are known to be activated in particular cancers directly or through dysregulation of upstream signaling elements.

KINASE INHIBITORS IN VETERINARY MEDICINE

Limited data exist on the clinical efficacy of small molecule inhibitors in veterinary medicine. In part, this is attributable to the high cost of treatment for affected patients, because there are currently no generic versions of available inhibitors. Additionally, targets for therapeutic intervention are not clearly defined for most canine cancers. Finally, toxicities not found in human beings are sometimes observed in dogs.

One target kinase known to be dysregulated in canine cancers is Kit. In approximately 25% to 30% of canine grade II and III mast cell tumors (MCTs), activating mutations resulting in constitutive activation in the absence of ligand binding are found in the juxtamembrane domain of Kit. These are associated with a higher risk of local recurrence and metastasis [61–63]. Although Gleevec effectively inhibits Kit signaling, it is known to induce hepatotoxicity in a proportion of treated dogs, thereby precluding its consistent use in canine patients. Other Kit inhibitors have been investigated, however.

A phase I trial exploring the safety and efficacy of SU11654, the veterinary counterpart to SUTENT, was completed [64]. Like SUTENT, SU11654 exhibits activity against the split kinase family (Kit, VEGFR, and PDGFR), and would therefore be predicted to have clinical activity in several types of cancer. Fifty-seven dogs with a variety of spontaneous neoplasms were enrolled in this study. Measurable objective responses were observed in 16 dogs for an overall response rate of 28% (16 of 57 dogs). Stable disease for longer than 10 weeks was seen in an additional 15 dogs for a resultant overall biologic activity rate of 54% (31 of 57 dogs). The highest response rate was observed in MCTs, which, as previously described, are often driven by aberrant Kit signaling. Responses were also noted in patients that had carcinomas, sarcomas, and multiple myeloma, however, likely secondary to SU11654 effects on VEGFR and PDGFR. This study provided the first evidence that multitargeted kinase inhibitors can exhibit broad activity against a variety of spontaneous malignancies in canine patients that had cancer. SU11654 is currently undergoing further clinical evaluation in dogs.

Recently, an open-label phase II study of a specific Kit inhibitor AB1010 (AB Science, Paris, France) was completed in dogs with grade II and III MCTs. Of 13 dogs treated, there were two complete responses, two partial responses, and stable disease in an additional 2 dogs; the drug was well tolerated (Axiak and colleagues, VCS 2006, personal communication, 2006). A randomized, double-blind, placebo-controlled, phase III study of AB1010 is ongoing in dogs with MCTs to confirm its clinical efficacy.

Other kinases currently under investigation for their potential role in canine cancers include EGFR and Met, among others. EGF stimulation of two malignant mammary lines could inhibit apoptosis induced by serum starvation or doxorubicin treatment (D. Thamm, personal communication, 2007). Furthermore, the cell lines demonstrated enhanced chemotaxis and VEGF production in response to EGF, and these were inhibited by ZD6474 (vandetanib, a small molecule inhibitor of VEGF, EGFR, and RET; Astra Zeneca). Studies from the author's laboratory have shown that a small molecule inhibitor of Met, PF2362376, blocks Met signaling in canine osteosarcoma cell lines and inhibits associated biologic activities, including scattering, migration, and colony formation; at higher doses, PF2362376 induces death of treated cells [65]. PF2362376 also blocked hepatocyte growth factor (HGF)–induced rescue of osteosarcoma cells after treatment with doxorubicin. These studies suggest that Met may be a relevant target for therapeutic intervention in canine osteosarcoma.

Although Gleevec may induce hepatotoxicity in dogs, it is apparently well tolerated in cats. A phase I clinical trial evaluating the toxicity of Gleevec was performed in 9 cats with a variety of tumors [66]. Doses of 10 to 15 mg/kg were well tolerated, with no evidence of hematologic toxicity and only mild gastrointestinal toxicity. Recently, a cat with systemic mastocytosis was treated with Gleevec at a dose of 10 mg/kg [67]. The cat exhibited a complete response to therapy at 5 weeks of treatment with no obvious toxicity. Interestingly, the malignant mast cells possessed a mutation in exon 8 of Kit (extracellular ligand binding domain). Mutations in this region of Kit have been described in human AML and are known to constitutive activation of Kit in the absence of ligand binding. Therefore, it is possible that the cat's mast cell disease was driven by Kit dysregulation in this instance, thus supporting the notion that inhibition of Kit signaling was responsible for the observed response to therapy.

Another feline tumor type that may benefit from Gleevec is vaccine-associated sarcoma (VAS). VAS cell lines were shown to express PDGFRβ, and Gleevec was shown to block PDGF-induced phosphorylation in these cells [68]. Additionally, Gleevec significantly inhibited the growth of VAS tumors in murine xenografts and reversed the protective effect of PDGF on doxorubicin- and carboplatin-induced growth inhibition. These studies support the notion that PDGFR may promote the growth and survival of VAS in vivo, and thus be an appropriate target for therapeutic intervention using targeted approaches.

HEAT SHOCK PROTEIN 90 INHIBITORS

Heat shock protein 90 (HSP90) is a member of a class of cellular proteins called chaperones. HSP90 forms a complex with additional proteins and acts to promote the correct conformation/folding, activity, intracellular localization, and turnover of a wide array of proteins involved in cell growth and survival (Fig. 2) [69–71]. Proteins that depend on correct HSP90 function (also known as "client" proteins) include Kit, Met, Akt, Raf, and Bcr-Abl, among others. The chaperone activity of HSP90 requires ATP, and inhibition of binding prevents the formation of the mature chaperone complex necessary for its intrinsic activity, eventually resulting in proteasome-dependent degradation of associated client proteins [72].

Although HSP90 does not seem to be mutated or subject to gene amplification in cancer cells, it is expressed at high levels in a wide range of human tumors [70,73]. This may be secondary to the general cellular stresses experienced by tumor cells, including abnormal microenvironment (hypoxia, acidosis, and nutrient deprivation) and abnormal cell signaling/cycling (dysregulated oncogenes/tumor suppressor genes). These stresses may make cancer cells more reliant on adequate HSP90 function, particularly in the setting of mutated client proteins, thereby enhancing the therapeutic selectivity of HSP90 inhibitors [74]. Furthermore, mutated client proteins exhibit conformational stress and require HSP90 activity to promote accurate folding. It has recently been shown that HSP90 extracted from tumor cells possesses 100-fold greater sensitivity to HSP90 inhibitors when compared with that isolated from normal cells [75]. Additional selectivity of HSP90 inhibitors for tumor cells may also exist through the downregulation of multiple client proteins in tumor cells that depend on these proteins for cell survival and proliferation (ie, Kit, Akt).

Given the potential ability of HSP90 inhibition to affect a variety of oncoproteins, significant effort has been directed at identifying small molecule inhibitors of this chaperone protein. Because the HSP90 complex requires the binding of ATP, most compounds have been developed to block the ATPase activity of the complex. The first inhibitor to enter human clinical trials was 17-AAG, a geldanamycin analogue. In phase I studies, activity was reported in melanoma, breast carcinoma, and prostate carcinoma, although this consisted primarily of prolonged stable disease [76,77]. 17-AAG possesses poor solubility, however, and results in clinical toxicities, including dehydration, diarrhea, and hepatotoxicity, that have precluded its practical use. A variety of newer HSP90 inhibitors have entered phase I clinical trials, including 17-DMAG and IP-504 (analogues of 17-AAG that are water-soluble and possess equal or greater activity), among others [71,78]. Early evidence suggests that these compounds induce less clinical toxicity while possessing equal or greater activity than 17-AAG.

Little is known regarding the status of HSP90 in canine and feline tumors. In two separate studies, expression of HSP90 was significantly increased in mammary tumors when compared with normal surrounding tissue [79,80]. The author's laboratory has been investigating the expression and potential role of HSP90 in canine MCTs. HSP90 was found to be expressed in normal canine bone marrow–derived mast cells and in malignant mast cell lines and malignant mast cells freshly isolated from MCTs. Treatment of the cell lines and malignant mast cells ex vivo with a novel HSP90 inhibitor (STA-9090; Synta, Synta Pharmaceuticals, Corp., Lexington, Massachusetts) resulted in rapid downregulation of Kit expression, ultimately resulting in apoptosis of treated cells (C. London, personal communication, 2007). These studies suggest that similar to the case of human cancers, particular canine cancers may depend on adequate HSP90 function to maintain client protein expression and sustain cell survival.

PROTEASOME INHIBITORS

Proteins in the cell are normally targeted for destruction (degradation) by a process known as ubiquitination, in which ubiquitin is conjugated to lysine residues of the protein. This process is part of the normal turnover of cellular proteins and is required to maintain homeostasis. The proteasome is an enzymatic complex that recognizes ubiquitin-labeled proteins and catalyzes their destruction [81–83]. Proteasomes are located in the cytoplasm and nucleus of the cell and consist of multiple subunits. In tumor cells, many proteins involved in tumorigenesis, such as cyclin-dependent kinase inhibitors, p53, and Bax, are regulated by ubiquitination and their degradation promotes cell survival and proliferation. Given the potential critical role of proteasome function in maintaining tumor cell integrity, several proteasome inhibitors are under development.

The first proteasome inhibitor to be developed, bortezomib (Velcade; Millenium Pharmaceuticals, Cambridge, Massachusetts), was initially designed to treat patients who had multiple myeloma, because it was observed that

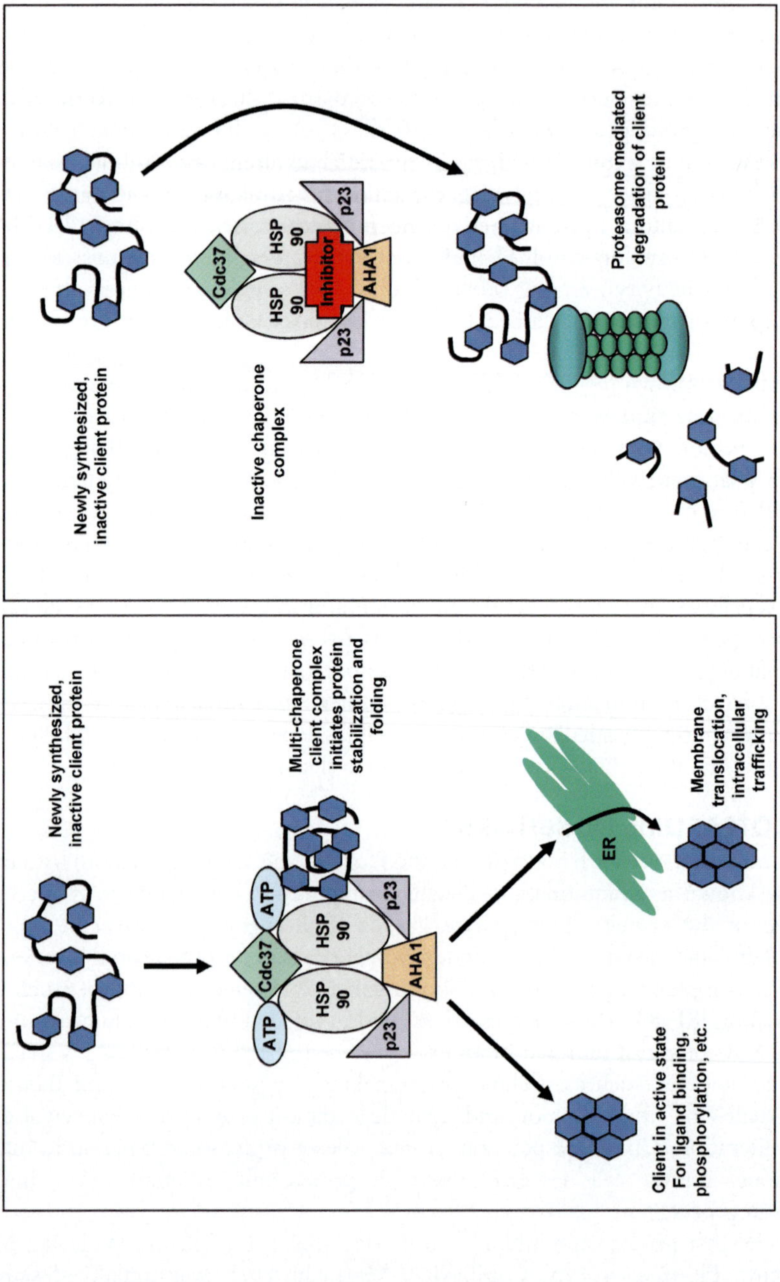
Newly synthesized, inactive client protein
ATP
Cdc37
HSP 90
HSP 90
ATP
p23
p23
AHA1
Multi-chaperone client complex initiates protein stabilization and folding
ER
Membrane translocation, intracellular trafficking
Client in active state For ligand binding, phosphorylation, etc.
Newly synthesized, inactive client protein
Inactive chaperone complex
Cdc37
HSP 90
HSP 90
Inhibitor
p23
p23
AHA1
Proteasome mediated degradation of client protein

normal plasma cells require proteasome activity for long-term survival [84]. As a single agent, significant clinical activity of bortezomib was noted in patients who had relapsed/refractory multiple myeloma, inducing overall response rates of 30% to 40%. When used in combination with chemotherapy, responses were noted in more than 50% of patients (reviewed by Nencioni and colleagues [85]). Based on these results, bortezomib was rapidly approved and is now used in combination with chemotherapy for previously untreated patients who have multiple myeloma, resulting in responses in greater than 75% of individuals.

Based on its excellent activity in multiple myeloma, bortezomib has been evaluated in several clinical trials for solid and hematologic malignancies. Although tremendous activity has not been noted in many tumor types, single-agent bortezimib does induce clinical responses in patients who have NSCLC and has recently been approved for relapsed/refractory mantle cell lymphoma [86,87]. A variety of novel proteasome inhibitors likely to possess better pharmacologic properties and less clinical toxicity than that observed with bortezomib are currently under development. The potential utility of bortezomib in veterinary patients that have cancer has not yet been investigated.

HISTONE DEACETYLASE INHIBITORS

DNA in cells is packaged in the form of what is termed a *nucleosome*, in which the DNA wraps around a nucleosomal core consisting of a complex of proteins termed *histones*. Packaged DNA is generally inaccessible to transcriptional machinery; thus, formation of the nucleosome helps to regulate gene expression. When histones are acetylated by histone acetyltransferase (HAT), their interactions with DNA are significantly diminished, inducing a conformational change that opens up the DNA, promoting the access of transcription and regulatory factors. This process is reversed by histone deacetylase (HDAC), which restores acetylation to the histones, thereby preventing transcription [88,89]. Evidence suggests that an imbalance of acetylation and deacetylation leads to dysregulation of cell differentiation, cell cycling, and cell survival, thereby contributing to carcinogenesis. Specifically, HDAC is frequently overexpressed in tumors, and several studies have shown that it prevents transcription of a variety of regulatory genes, such as the cell cycle inhibitor p21 and p53 [88,90]. Furthermore, aberrant HDAC activity has been associated with the upregulation of genes that contribute to tumorigenesis, including VEGF and HIF1α [91].

Fig. 2. HSP90 and client protein activation. (*Left*) Newly synthesized client proteins interact with the multichaperone complex containing HSP90, p23, CDC37, AHA1, and ATPase activity, resulting in the inhibition of aggregation, appropriate folding of the client protein enabling its biologic function, and intracellular trafficking, particularly across the endoplasmic reticulum (ER). (*Right*) HSP90 inhibitors block formation of the active multichaperone complex, thereby preventing client protein folding, ultimately resulting in proteasome-mediated degradation of the client protein.

Given its increasingly important role in neoplastic transformation and gene regulation, HDAC has been identified as an important target for therapeutic intervention. A variety of HDAC inhibitors have been investigated, and several are now in human clinical trials. Perhaps the best known of these is suberolyanilide hydroxamic acid (SAHA), which has been tested extensively in animal models of cancer [91,92]. Although micromolar concentrations of SAHA are required for effective inhibition of HDAC in vivo, the drug is generally well tolerated.

In a phase I clinical trial, SAHA was administered intravenously to patients who had tumors refractory to standard treatments. The dose-limiting toxicity was thrombocytopenia and neutropenia in the patients who had hematologic but not solid tumors. Other toxicities included fatigue, diarrhea, and anorexia. Activity was noted across a broad range of tumor types, including thyroid carcinoma, mesothelioma, and lymphoma [93]. An oral preparation has been developed that has good oral bioavailability and pharmacokinetics [94]. Recently, a phase II study of refractory cutaneous T-cell lymphoma was completed, and 21% of treated patients experienced partial responses [95]. Given these encouraging results, there are now more than 30 ongoing SAHA clinical trials as a single agent or in combination with other agents.

There is little known about the role of HDAC in veterinary tumors because no clinical trials have been performed to date. Work in vitro has shown some promising activity against canine tumor cell lines, however. A novel phenylbutyrate-based HDAC inhibitor, OSU-HDAC42, was found to be effective against canine lymphoma, osteosarcoma, mast cell, and transitional cell carcinoma cell lines, reducing cell viability and inducing apoptosis (W. Kisseberth, personal communication, 2007). When compared with SAHA, OSU-HDAC42 demonstrated enhanced toxicity at lower concentrations of drug.

Another line of study involves the combination of valproic acid (VPA; also an HDAC inhibitor) with chemotherapy to enhance the chemosensitivity of osteosarcoma cells. Early data suggest that preincubation of canine osteosarcoma cell lines with VPA before exposure to doxorubicin markedly potentiates apoptosis in treated cells. Furthermore, mice bearing canine osteosarcoma xenografts treated with VPA and doxorubicin exhibited significant tumor growth inhibition and prolongation of survival when compared with mice treated with either drug alone (D. Thamm, personal communication, 2007). These studies support the notion that similar to the case in human beings, HDAC inhibitors are likely to be of benefit for canine patients, particularly when these drugs are used in combination therapies.

SUMMARY

Small molecule inhibitors of dysregulated cellular proteins have not only helped to dissect the biology of cancer but have provided a new and sometimes extremely effective approach to its treatment. In veterinary as well as human oncology, challenges ahead lie in identifying appropriate targets for therapeutic intervention and in combining targeted therapeutics with standard treatment modalities, such as radiation and chemotherapy.

References

[1] London CA. Kinase inhibitors in cancer therapy. Veterinary and Comparative Oncology 2004;2(4):177-93.
[2] Zwick E, Bange J, Ullrich A. Receptor tyrosine kinases as targets for anticancer drugs. Trends Mol Med 2002;8(1):17-23.
[3] Madhusudan S, Ganesan TS. Tyrosine kinase inhibitors in cancer therapy. Clin Biochem 2004;37(7):618-35.
[4] Ma PC, Maulik G, Christensen J, et al. c-Met: structure, functions and potential for therapeutic inhibition. Cancer Metastasis Rev 2003;22(4):309-25.
[5] Laskin JJ, Sandler AB. Epidermal growth factor receptor: a promising target in solid tumours. Cancer Treat Rev 2004;30(1):1-17.
[6] Fletcher JA. Role of KIT and platelet-derived growth factor receptors as oncoproteins. Semin Oncol 2004;31(2 Suppl 6):4-11.
[7] Neubauer A, Burchert A, Maiwald C, et al. Recent progress on the role of Axl, a receptor tyrosine kinase, in malignant transformation of myeloid leukemias. Leuk Lymphoma 1997; 25(1-2):91-6.
[8] Thurston G, Gale NW. Vascular endothelial growth factor and other signaling pathways in developmental and pathologic angiogenesis. Int J Hematol 2004;80(1):7-20.
[9] Eskens FA. Angiogenesis inhibitors in clinical development; where are we now and where are we going? Br J Cancer 2004;90(1):1-7.
[10] Cherrington JM, Strawn LM, Shawver LK. New paradigms for the treatment of cancer: the role of anti-angiogenesis agents. Adv Cancer Res 2000;79:1-38.
[11] McCarty MF, Liu W, Fan F, et al. Promises and pitfalls of anti-angiogenic therapy in clinical trials. Trends Mol Med 2003;9(2):53-8.
[12] Thurston G. Role of angiopoietins and tie receptor tyrosine kinases in angiogenesis and lymphangiogenesis. Cell Tissue Res 2003;314(1):61-8.
[13] Johnson GL, Lapadat R. Mitogen-activated protein kinase pathways mediated by ERK, JNK, and p38 protein kinases. Science 2002;298(5600):1911-2.
[14] Downward J. Targeting RAS signalling pathways in cancer therapy. Nat Rev Cancer 2003;3(1):11-22.
[15] Davies H, Bignell GR, Cox C, et al. Mutations of the BRAF gene in human cancer. Nature 2002;417(6892):949-54.
[16] Kumar R, Angelini S, Snellman E, et al. BRAF mutations are common somatic events in melanocytic nevi. J Invest Dermatol 2004;122(2):342-8.
[17] Mercer KE, Pritchard CA. Raf proteins and cancer: B-Raf is identified as a mutational target. Biochim Biophys Acta 2003;1653(1):25-40.
[18] Fresno Vara JA, Casado E, de Castro J, et al. PI3K/Akt signalling pathway and cancer. Cancer Treat Rev 2004;30(2):193-204.
[19] Franke TF, Hornik CP, Segev L, et al. PI3K/Akt and apoptosis: size matters. Oncogene 2003;22(56):8983-98.
[20] Mitsiades CS, Mitsiades N, Koutsilieris M. The Akt pathway: molecular targets for anticancer drug development. Curr Cancer Drug Targets 2004;4(3):235-56.
[21] Chian R, Young S, Danilkovitch-Miagkova A, et al. PI3 kinase mediates transformation of hematopoietic cells by the V816 c-kit mutant. Blood 2001;98(5):1365-73.
[22] Shayesteh L, Lu Y, Kuo WL, et al. PIK3CA is implicated as an oncogene in ovarian cancer. Nat Genet 1999;21(1):99-102.
[23] Cheng JQ, Ruggeri B, Klein WM, et al. Amplification of AKT2 in human pancreatic cells and inhibition of AKT2 expression and tumorigenicity by antisense RNA. Proc Natl Acad Sci USA 1996;93(8):3636-41.

[24] Bellacosa A, de Feo D, Godwin AK, et al. Molecular alterations of the AKT2 oncogene in ovarian and breast carcinomas. Int J Cancer 1995;64(4):280–5.
[25] Simpson L, Parsons R. PTEN: life as a tumor suppressor. Exp Cell Res 2001;264(1):29–41.
[26] Weng LP, Smith WM, Dahia PL, et al. PTEN suppresses breast cancer cell growth by phosphatase activity-dependent G1 arrest followed by cell death. Cancer Res 1999;59(22): 5808–14.
[27] Shchemelinin I, Sefc L, Necas E. Protein kinases, their function and implication in cancer and other diseases. Folia Biol (Praha) 2006;52(3):81–100.
[28] Wanebo HJ, Argiris A, Bergsland E, et al. Targeting growth factors and angiogenesis; using small molecules in malignancy. Cancer Metastasis Rev 2006;25(2):279–92.
[29] Shchemelinin I, Sefc L, Necas E. Protein kinase inhibitors. Folia Biol (Praha) 2006;52(4): 137–48.
[30] Wakeling AE. Inhibitors of growth factor signalling. Endocr Relat Cancer 2005;12(Suppl 1):S183–7.
[31] Alvarez RH, Kantarjian H, Cortes JE. The biology of chronic myelogenous leukemia: implications for imatinib therapy. Semin Hematol 2007;44(1 Suppl 1):S4–14.
[32] Moen MD, McKeage K, Plosker GL, et al. Imatinib: a review of its use in chronic myeloid leukaemia. Drugs 2007;67(2):299–320.
[33] Mauro MJ, Druker BJ. STI571: targeting BCR-ABL as therapy for CML. Oncologist 2001; 6(3):233–8.
[34] Kantarjian H, Sawyers C, Hochhaus A, et al. Hematologic and cytogenetic responses to imatinib mesylate in chronic myelogenous leukemia. N Engl J Med 2002;346(9):645–52.
[35] Beham-Schmid C, Apfelbeck U, Sill H, et al. Treatment of chronic myelogenous leukemia with the tyrosine kinase inhibitor STI571 results in marked regression of bone marrow fibrosis. Blood 2002;99(1):381–3.
[36] Druker BJ, Talpaz M, Resta DJ, et al. Efficacy and safety of a specific inhibitor of the BCR-ABL tyrosine kinase in chronic myeloid leukemia. N Engl J Med 2001;344(14):1031–7.
[37] Druker BJ, Sawyers CL, Kantarjian H, et al. Activity of a specific inhibitor of the BCR-ABL tyrosine kinase in the blast crisis of chronic myeloid leukemia and acute lymphoblastic leukemia with the Philadelphia chromosome. N Engl J Med 2001;344(14):1038–42.
[38] Sawyers CL. Rational therapeutic intervention in cancer: kinases as drug targets. Curr Opin Genet Dev 2002;12(1):111–5.
[39] Nardi V, Azam M, Daley GQ. Mechanisms and implications of imatinib resistance mutations in BCR-ABL. Curr Opin Hematol 2004;11(1):35–43.
[40] Weisberg E, Griffin JD. Resistance to imatinib (Glivec): update on clinical mechanisms. Drug Resist Updat 2003;6(5):231–8.
[41] Galli SJ, Zsebo KM, Geissler EN. The kit ligand, stem cell factor. Adv Immunol 1994;55: 1–95.
[42] Gotlib J. KIT mutations in mastocytosis and their potential as therapeutic targets. Immunol Allergy Clin North Am 2006;26(3):575–92.
[43] Advani AS. C-kit as a target in the treatment of acute myelogenous leukemia. Curr Hematol Rep 2005;4(1):51–8.
[44] Lasota J, Miettinen M. KIT and PDGFRA mutations in gastrointestinal stromal tumors (GISTs). Semin Diagn Pathol 2006;23(2):91–102.
[45] Siddiqui MA, Scott LJ. Imatinib: a review of its use in the management of gastrointestinal stromal tumours. Drugs 2007;67(5):805–20.
[46] Duffaud F, Blay JY. Gastrointestinal stromal tumors: biology and treatment. Oncology 2003;65(3):187–97.
[47] Heinrich MC, Rubin BP, Longley BJ, et al. Biology and genetic aspects of gastrointestinal stromal tumors: KIT activation and cytogenetic alterations. Hum Pathol 2002;33(5):484–95, t&artType=abs&id=ahupa0330484&target=.
[48] Miettinen M, Sarlomo-Rikala M, Lasota J. Gastrointestinal stromal tumors: recent advances in understanding of their biology. Hum Pathol 1999;30(10):1213–20.

[49] Miettinen M, Sarlomo-Rikala M, Lasota J. Gastrointestinal stromal tumours. Ann Chir Gynaecol 1998;87(4):278–81.
[50] Heinrich MC, Corless CL, Duensing A, et al. PDGFRA activating mutations in gastrointestinal stromal tumors. Science 2003;299(5607):708–10.
[51] Chow LQ, Eckhardt SG. Sunitinib: from rational design to clinical efficacy. J Clin Oncol 2007;25(7):884–96.
[52] Ranson M, Wardell S. Gefitinib, a novel, orally administered agent for the treatment of cancer. J Clin Pharm Ther 2004;29(2):95–103.
[53] Roskoski R Jr. The ErbB/HER receptor protein-tyrosine kinases and cancer. Biochem Biophys Res Commun 2004;319(1):1–11.
[54] Lynch TJ, Bell DW, Sordella R, et al. Activating mutations in the epidermal growth factor receptor underlying responsiveness of non-small-cell lung cancer to gefitinib. N Engl J Med 2004;350(21):2129–39.
[55] Wan PT, Garnett MJ, Roe SM, et al. Mechanism of activation of the RAF-ERK signaling pathway by oncogenic mutations of B-RAF. Cell 2004;116(6):855–67.
[56] Dhillon AS, Kolch W. Oncogenic B-Raf mutations: crystal clear at last. Cancer Cell 2004;5(4):303–4.
[57] Hotte SJ, Hirte HW. BAY 43-9006: early clinical data in patients with advanced solid malignancies. Curr Pharm Des 2002;8(25):2249–53.
[58] Lyons JF, Wilhelm S, Hibner B, et al. Discovery of a novel Raf kinase inhibitor. Endocr Relat Cancer 2001;8(3):219–25.
[59] Lee JT, McCubrey JA. BAY-43-9006 Bayer/Onyx. Curr Opin Investig Drugs 2003;4(6):757–63.
[60] Flaherty KT. Sorafenib in renal cell carcinoma. Clin Cancer Res 2007;13(2 Pt 2):747S–52S.
[61] Zemke D, Yamini B, Yuzbasiyan-Gurkan V. Mutations in the juxtamembrane domain of c-KIT are associated with higher grade mast cell tumors in dogs. Vet Pathol 2002;39(5):529–35.
[62] Downing S, Chien MB, Kass PH, et al. Prevalence and importance of internal tandem duplications in exons 11 and 12 of c-kit in mast cell tumors of dogs. Am J Vet Res 2002;63:1718–23.
[63] London CA, Galli SJ, Yuuki T, et al. Spontaneous canine mast cell tumors express tandem duplications in the proto-oncogene c-kit. Exp Hematol 1999;27:689–97.
[64] London CA, Hannah AL, Zadovoskaya R, et al. Phase I dose-escalating study of SU11654, a small molecule receptor tyrosine kinase inhibitor, in dogs with spontaneous malignancies. Clin Cancer Res 2003;9(7):2755–68.
[65] Liao AT, McCleese J, Kamerling S, et al. A novel small molecule Met inhibitor, PF2362376, exhibits biological activity against canine osteosarcoma. Veterinary and Comparative Oncology, in press.
[66] Lachowicz JL, Post GS, Brodsky E. A phase I clinical trial evaluating imatinib mesylate (Gleevec) in tumor-bearing cats. J Vet Intern Med 2005;19(6):860–4.
[67] Isotani M, Tamura K, Yagihara H, et al. Identification of a c-kit exon 8 internal tandem duplication in a feline mast cell tumor case and its favorable response to the tyrosine kinase inhibitor imatinib mesylate. Vet Immunol Immunopathol 2006;114(1–2):168–72.
[68] Katayama R, Huelsmeyer MK, Marr AK, et al. Imatinib mesylate inhibits platelet-derived growth factor activity and increases chemosensitivity in feline vaccine-associated sarcoma. Cancer Chemother Pharmacol 2004;54(1):25–33.
[69] Whitesell L, Lindquist SL. HSP90 and the chaperoning of cancer. Nat Rev Cancer 2005;5(10):761–72.
[70] Maloney A, Workman P. HSP90 as a new therapeutic target for cancer therapy: the story unfolds. Expert Opin Biol Ther 2002;2(1):3–24.
[71] Powers MV, Workman P. Targeting of multiple signalling pathways by heat shock protein 90 molecular chaperone inhibitors. Endocr Relat Cancer 2006;13(Suppl 1):S125–35.
[72] Connell P, Ballinger CA, Jiang J, et al. The co-chaperone CHIP regulates protein triage decisions mediated by heat-shock proteins. Nat Cell Biol 2001;3(1):93–6.

[73] Sreedhar AS, Kalmar E, Csermely P, et al. Hsp90 isoforms: functions, expression and clinical importance. FEBS Lett 2004;562(1–3):11–5.
[74] Whitesell L, Bagatell R, Falsey R. The stress response: implications for the clinical development of Hsp90 inhibitors. Curr Cancer Drug Targets 2003;3(5):349–58.
[75] Kamal A, Thao L, Sensintaffar J, et al. A high-affinity conformation of Hsp90 confers tumour selectivity on Hsp90 inhibitors. Nature 2003;425(6956):407–10.
[76] Banerji U, O'Donnell A, Scurr M, et al. Phase I pharmacokinetic and pharmacodynamic study of 17-allylamino, 17-demethoxygeldanamycin in patients with advanced malignancies. J Clin Oncol 2005;23(18):4152–61.
[77] Pacey S, Banerji U, Judson I, et al. Hsp90 inhibitors in the clinic. Handb Exp Pharmacol 2006;172:331–58.
[78] Hollingshead M, Alley M, Burger AM, et al. In vivo antitumor efficacy of 17-DMAG (17-dimethylaminoethylamino-17-demethoxygeldanamycin hydrochloride), a water-soluble geldanamycin derivative. Cancer Chemother Pharmacol 2005;56(2):115–25.
[79] Kumaraguruparan R, Karunagaran D, Balachandran C, et al. Of humans and canines: a comparative evaluation of heat shock and apoptosis-associated proteins in mammary tumors. Clin Chim Acta 2006;365(1–2):168–76.
[80] Romanucci M, Marinelli A, Sarli G, et al. Heat shock protein expression in canine malignant mammary tumours. BMC Cancer 2006;6:171.
[81] Adams J. The development of proteasome inhibitors as anticancer drugs. Cancer Cell 2004;5(5):417–21.
[82] Adams J. The proteasome: a suitable antineoplastic target. Nat Rev Cancer 2004;4(5):349–60.
[83] Mani A, Gelmann EP. The ubiquitin-proteasome pathway and its role in cancer. J Clin Oncol 2005;23(21):4776–89.
[84] Cenci S, Mezghrani A, Cascio P, et al. Progressively impaired proteasomal capacity during terminal plasma cell differentiation. EMBO J 2006;25(5):1104–13.
[85] Nencioni A, Grunebach F, Patrone F, et al. Proteasome inhibitors: antitumor effects and beyond. Leukemia 2007;21(1):30–6.
[86] Scagliotti G. Proteasome inhibitors in lung cancer. Crit Rev Oncol Hematol 2006;58(3):177–89.
[87] Fisher RI, Bernstein SH, Kahl BS, et al. Multicenter phase II study of bortezomib in patients with relapsed or refractory mantle cell lymphoma. J Clin Oncol 2006;24(30):4867–74.
[88] Carey N, La Thangue NB. Histone deacetylase inhibitors: gathering pace. Curr Opin Pharmacol 2006;6(4):369–75.
[89] Kim DH, Kim M, Kwon HJ. Histone deacetylase in carcinogenesis and its inhibitors as anticancer agents. J Biochem Mol Biol 2003;36(1):110–9.
[90] Marks PA, Jiang X. Histone deacetylase inhibitors in programmed cell death and cancer therapy. Cell Cycle 2005;4(4):549–51.
[91] Marks PA. Discovery and development of SAHA as an anticancer agent. Oncogene 2007;26(9):1351–6.
[92] Kelly WK, Marks PA. Drug insight: histone deacetylase inhibitors—development of the new targeted anticancer agent suberoylanilide hydroxamic acid. Nat Clin Pract Oncol 2005;2(3):150–7.
[93] Kelly WK, Richon VM, O'Connor O, et al. Phase I clinical trial of histone deacetylase inhibitor: suberoylanilide hydroxamic acid administered intravenously. Clin Cancer Res 2003;9(10 Pt 1):3578–88.
[94] Kelly WK, O'Connor OA, Krug LM, et al. Phase I study of an oral histone deacetylase inhibitor, suberoylanilide hydroxamic acid, in patients with advanced cancer. J Clin Oncol 2005;23(17):3923–31.
[95] Duvic M, Talpur R, Ni X, et al. Phase 2 trial of oral vorinostat (suberoylanilide hydroxamic acid, SAHA) for refractory cutaneous T-cell lymphoma (CTCL). Blood 2007;109(1):31–9.

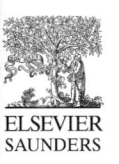

Cancer Immunotherapy for the Veterinary Patient

Barbara J. Biller, DVM, PhD

Department of Clinical Sciences, College of Veterinary Medicine and Biomedical Sciences, Colorado State University, James L. Voss Veterinary Teaching Hospital, 300 West Drake Road, Fort Collins, CO 80523-1620, USA

Most cancer immunotherapeutics are designed to activate cellular components of the antitumor immune response or selectively target critical features of the tumor itself. In this article, the author focuses on immunotherapeutics that stimulate immunity in general (nonspecific tumor immunotherapy) and some of the tumor-specific approaches, such as the use of monoclonal antibodies (mAbs) and immunotoxins. The discussion is centered on therapies currently available to the veterinary oncology patient or those that are undergoing evaluation in preclinical or early-phase clinical trials. Tumor vaccines are discussed in more detail elsewhere in this issue.

NONSPECIFIC TUMOR IMMUNOTHERAPY

In the late 1800s, William Coley, a surgeon, observed that patients having cancer and developing secondary bacterial infections often survived longer than those without infection [1,2]. Reasoning that stimulation of the immune system might slow tumor growth, Coley developed a bacterial "vaccine" consisting of killed cultures of *Streptococcus pyogenes* and *Serratia marcescens* ("Coley's toxins") that he used to treat people with inoperable bone and soft tissue sarcomas. Despite remarkable success in many patients, including complete and durable tumor remissions, the frequent occurrence of side effects and considerable skepticism from other physicians led to discontinuation of this approach [1]. Coley's work, however, laid the foundation for nonspecific modulation of the immune response as an approach to the treatment of cancer.

The goal of nonspecific immunotherapy is to engage the innate and adaptive arms of the immune response in recognition and attack of malignant cells. In general, better stimulation of the innate component, driven primarily by professional antigen-presenting cells, such as dendritic cells (DCs) and macrophages, leads to more effective T- and B-cell–mediated adaptive immune responses.

E-mail address: bbiller@colostate.edu

Therefore, many of the nonspecific immunotherapeutics (also known as biologic response modifiers) are efficient activators of innate immunity.

Biologic Response Modifiers

Bacillus of Calmette and Guérin and Mycobacterial Cell Wall–DNA Complex

The bacillus of Calmette and Guérin (BCG), a modified strain of *Mycobacterium bovis*, initially developed as a vaccine for tuberculosis in the early twentieth century, is an extension of Coley's work that is still in use today. Infusion of BCG into the bladder is one of the most successful forms of treatment for superficial bladder cancer in human patients. BCG is more effective than chemotherapy, especially in treating and preventing relapse of noninvasive transitional cell carcinoma (TCC) [3,4]. Although the mechanism for its antitumor effects are not completely understood, BCG stimulates a T helper type 1 (Th1) immune response mediated primarily by the production of inflammatory cytokines, such as interferon (IFN)-γ, IFNα, and interleukin (IL)-2. This response results in T-cell–mediated cytotoxicity of tumor cells and the induction of long-lived memory T cells that provide protection from relapsing disease [5,6].

Although BCG demonstrates antitumor efficacy against canine TCC in vitro and can be instilled into the bladder without induction of significant toxicity, it is rarely used as a form of cancer treatment because of the frequently invasive nature of canine TCC [7,8]. Intralesional BCG has been used successfully to treat ocular squamous cell carcinoma in cattle and sarcoids in horses; however, studies evaluating the efficacy of intralesional and intravenous BCG therapy in dogs with mammary tumors or osteosarcoma (OSA) have been disappointing [9,10].

A recent clinical trial in dogs with mast cell tumors (MCTs) suggests that BCG may be more useful when combined with other immunotherapeutics. When administered subcutaneously along with human chorionic gonadotropin (hCG), a compound that has immunomodulatory and antitumor effects against various human malignancies, BCG/hCG therapy was found to be as effective as standard vinblastine chemotherapy for control of grade II or III MCT [11]. In this large, randomized, phase II trial, significantly less toxicity was observed in the immunotherapy group compared with dogs treated with single-agent vinblastine.

A related compound known as mycobacterial cell wall–DNA complex (MCC) has also been assessed as an immunotherapeutic agent in dogs [12]. MCC is a bifunctional anticancer agent that induces tumor cell apoptosis and stimulates inflammatory cytokine production in a manner similar to BCG [13]. In vitro, MCC inhibits proliferation and induces apoptosis in several canine TCC and OSA cell lines [12,14]. Interestingly, apoptotic activity was enhanced by addition of piroxicam or pamidronate to TCC or OSA cultures, respectively, suggesting that the antitumor effects of MCC were synergistic with other forms of therapy. Clinical experience with MCC in dogs is limited; in a pilot study of dogs with TCC, two dogs had small reductions in tumor volume with no treatment-related toxicities [12]. Unfortunately, clinical trials with MCC are currently limited by difficulties in the manufacturing process of the drug (D. Knapp, West Lafayette, IN, personal communication, 2007).

Liposome-encapsulated muramyl tripeptide
Similar to the biologic response modifier MCC, muramyl tripeptide phosphatidylethanolamine (MTP-PE) is also derived from a portion of the *Mycobacterium* cell wall. Enclosure of MTP-PE within a liposome enables efficient uptake by monocytes and macrophages, greatly increasing the tumoricidal abilities of these cells and stimulating a cascade of innate and adaptive antitumor immune responses in the host. The combined product is known as liposome-encapsulated muramyl tripeptide (L-MTP-PE) and has been evaluated in human and veterinary clinical trials. In people, L-MTP-PE is most frequently used to treat high-grade and recurrent pediatric OSA [15]. In a recently completed phase III clinical trial, children treated with L-MTP-PE in combination with multidrug chemotherapy in the adjuvant setting had significantly higher survival and disease-free intervals than patients receiving chemotherapy alone [15].

In veterinary oncology, L-MTP-PE has been evaluated in clinical trials for cats with mammary adenocarcinoma and dogs with OSA, hemangiosarcoma (HSA), melanoma, and mammary adenocarcinoma [16–21]. L-MTP-PE therapy seems to be most effective for dogs with appendicular OSA; when dogs were randomized to receive L-MTP-PE after four doses of cisplatin (70 mg/m^2 every 4 weeks), median survival times of 14.4 months were observed compared with 10 months in dogs receiving cisplatin alone ($P<.05$) [18]. Dogs receiving L-MTP-PE were also less likely to develop metastatic disease (73% versus 93%) than dogs treated with chemotherapy alone.

L-MTP-PE also demonstrates antitumor activity in commonly occurring canine malignancies, such as HSA and oral melanoma. In a study of dogs with splenic HSA, patients receiving L-MTP-PE in combination with adjuvant doxorubicin/cyclophosphamide demonstrated a significantly increased survival time of 9 months compared with 5.7 months for dogs treated with chemotherapy alone [17]. In dogs with stage I oral melanoma, adjuvant therapy with L-MTP-PE, used as a single agent or combined with recombinant canine granulocyte macrophage colony-stimulating factor (rcGM-CSF), extended survival times compared with dogs undergoing surgery alone [20]. This study, however, did not demonstrate any therapeutic advantage of rcGM-CSF over single-agent L-MTP-PE therapy.

Unfortunately, the availability of L-MTP-PE is currently limited. L-MTP-PE (also known as Mepact) has recently received orphan drug status in Europe and the United States; regulatory approval for its use in human beings is expected in late 2007 or early 2008. The drug is expected to be available for off-label use by veterinarians but is initially likely to be cost-prohibitive.

Liposome-DNA complexes
Activation of DCs, the most potent of the antigen-presenting cells, is a crucial aspect in the generation of effective antitumor immunity. Bacterial DNA, which contains repeated segments of the bases cystine and guanine (or CpG motifs), is

a strong activator of innate immunity; these responses are markedly enhanced when the DNA is complexed to cationic liposomes [22,23]. Studies of liposome-DNA complex (LDC) immunotherapy in mouse tumor models have shown induction of strong antitumor activity, which seems to be mediated largely through stimulation of natural killer (NK) cell activity; DC activation; and release of proinflammatory cytokines, such as type I IFNs, IL-12, and IFNγ [22,24–26].

The author's laboratory has been investigating LDC immunotherapy in dogs with cancer. In a nonrandomized phase I/II trial in dogs with melanoma or HSA, LDC combined with an allogeneic tumor cell lysate was administered to client-owned dogs once every 2 weeks for five treatments and then once monthly for at least 3 months [27,28]. Toxicity was minimal, with only 6 of 75 dogs experiencing nausea, transient fever, or mild to moderate abdominal pain. Determination of overall efficacy was complicated by the use of multiple treatment protocols in addition to LDC immunotherapy, but the median survival of dogs with HSA was significantly longer than that of a control population. No increase in disease-free interval or survival was found for dogs with melanoma. Additional studies evaluating the use of LDC as single-agent therapy and in combination with other treatment modalities, such as radiation and chemotherapy, are ongoing.

Another potential application of LDC therapy is systemic gene delivery. This approach is particularly attractive in targeting pulmonary tumors, because most gene expression has been shown to occur in the lungs after intravenous administration of LDC [29]. A study by Dow and colleagues [30] demonstrated the feasibility of this approach in dogs with pulmonary metastatic OSC; intravenous delivery of LDC encoding the IL-2 gene elicited potent immune activation and NK cell activity and was associated with a significant increase in survival times compared with historical controls. In dogs with soft tissue sarcoma, intravenous infusions of LDC containing canine endostatin DNA inhibited tumor angiogenesis and resulted in objective tumor responses or stable disease for 8 of 12 dogs receiving the therapy [31].

Oncolytic viruses

Viruses that preferentially replicate within and lyse tumor cells are referred to as oncolytic. The replication cycle of many viruses uses the same cellular pathways that are frequently altered in malignant cells [32]. Because they are tumor-selective, oncolytic viruses offer an attractive approach for targeted delivery of genes, drugs, and cytokines to malignant cells. They are also capable of direct tumor cell killing and can further enhance antitumor immunity through stimulation of host innate and adaptive immune responses.

The canine distemper virus (CDV), an enveloped morbillivirus within the family Paramyxoviridae, is emerging as a promising immunotherapeutic agent for the treatment of canine lymphoma. Suter and colleagues [33] recently demonstrated selective binding of attenuated CDV to CD46 and CD150, two cell membrane proteins that are commonly overexpressed on malignant lymphocytes. CDV binding to either of these cell surface markers led to CDV infection, followed by lysis of the neoplastic cells. Apoptosis of CD46- or CD150-expressing immortalized lymphoid cell lines and freshly isolated neoplastic lymphocytes from tumor-bearing dogs were observed, suggesting the possibility of using attenuated CDV to treat dogs with lymphoma.

The adenoviruses are also being investigated in veterinary oncology and are especially attractive because of their potential to mediate gene transfer and tumor cell lysis. A promising candidate is the canine adenovirus type 2 (CAV2), which has recently been shown to deliver numerous genes to canine OSA tumors efficiently in vitro and in vivo [34,35]. In the OSA model, CAV2 expression can be controlled using an osteocalcin promoter, thus enabling control of oncolytic viral replication once gene delivery has occurred [36].

Cytokine Therapy
Interleukin-2
The observation that treatment of mice that had disseminated cancer with IL-2 induced complete tumor regression stimulated tremendous interest in the 1980s in the potential use of recombinant cytokine therapy in people with advanced malignancies [37]. IL-2 elicits a cascade of immunomodulatory effects, including T-cell activation and expansion, stimulation of antigen-presenting cells, proinflammatory cytokine secretion, and augmentation of NK and lymphokine-activated killer (LAK) cell function. Unfortunately, however, the dramatic antitumor and immunostimulatory properties of IL-2 therapy are also associated with significant side effects, especially when IL-2 is administered intravenously or in high doses.

To take advantage of the antitumor activities of IL-2 while avoiding its toxicity, many alternative methods of IL-2 delivery have been evaluated, including intratumor injection, adenoviral-mediated gene delivery, and the use of antibody–IL-2 fusion proteins that specifically target neoplastic cells. Systemic IL-2 therapy is now usually combined with other treatment modalities, such as chemotherapy, radiation therapy, and other forms of immunotherapy, to increase the antitumor effectiveness of the primary treatment and to permit lower doses of IL-2.

An intriguing application of IL-2 therapy in veterinary oncology is targeting of IL-2 to the lungs through liposome encapsulation. In addition to administration of intravenous LDC–IL-2 as described previously, liposome-encapsulated IL-2 can be delivered by nebulization. This approach has been evaluated in dogs with metastatic pulmonary OSC and primary lung carcinoma. In a pilot study by Khanna and colleagues [38], inhalational liposome–IL-2 therapy was well tolerated and was not associated with significant toxicity. Two of four dogs with metastatic pulmonary OSA had complete regression of metastases; regression was stable for more than 12 months in one dog and for more than 20 months in the other. This study initiated multiple clinical trials in people with pulmonary metastatic disease; when used to treat pulmonary metastases of renal cell carcinoma, for example, objective response rates of

14% to 30% and increased progression-free and overall survival times were reported [39].

Interleukin-12

Like IL-2, IL-12 has pronounced stimulatory effects on the innate and adaptive arms of the immune response. In addition, IL-12 is a potent antiangiogenic cytokine, and can therefore slow tumor growth through immunomodulatory and antiangiogenic effects. As is the case for many cytokines, IL-12 exhibits high sequence homology between species [40,41]. Although IL-12 has been sequenced and cloned in the dog, human recombinant interleukin-12 (hrIL-12) has also been found to cross-react with the canine IL-12 receptor and is more readily available [40,42].

The immunostimulatory and antiangiogenic potential of IL-12 therapy is currently being investigated in the veterinary field. For example, Akhtar and colleagues [43] developed a method to target IL-12 to a canine HSA tumor cell line by creating a fusion protein with an integrin adhesion molecule expressed on immature endothelial cells. Targeted IL-12 therapy was not only effective in slowing the growth of canine HSA tumors engrafted onto mice but permitted the use of a lower dose of the cytokine than that needed to demonstrate the antiangiogenic activity of IL-12 alone. These results support further evaluation of targeted IL-12 therapy as a treatment approach to dogs with localized HSA, such as those with the subcutaneous form of the disease.

IL-12 is also under investigation for its use in cancer gene therapy. In cats undergoing radiation therapy for soft tissue sarcoma, IL-12 gene expression was coupled to a heat-inducible promoter; this construct was then administered by intratumoral injection and followed with tumor hyperthermia to induce the expression of IL-12 [44]. The investigators found that although feline IL-12 mRNA was present in high levels within tumor tissue, IFNγ mRNA expression was low, suggesting that stimulation of local antitumor immunity was minimal. Although this treatment approach is presently constrained by the limited availability of hyperthermia, the trial demonstrated the feasibility and safety of tumor-targeted IL-12 gene expression in cats.

Tumor necrosis factor-α

Tumor necrosis factor-α (TNFα) was the first member of the large TNF and TNF-receptor superfamily of proteins to be identified. Although nearly all cells in the body can produce TNFα in response to inflammatory stimuli, production by macrophages and monocytes is the primary source. TNFα was initially identified based on its ability to induce apoptosis in tumor cell lines in vitro. Its utility as an immunotherapy agent, however, stems from the important role of this proinflammatory cytokine in activation of immune responses and selective cytotoxic effects on tumor endothelial cells and angiogenic vessels [45,46]. Similar to the other cytokines discussed previously, systemic administration of TNFα is associated with significant toxicity; therefore, tumor-targeted therapy seems to be most promising.

One such approach is delivery of TNFα within a bacteriophage. Filamentous bacteriophages are attractive vehicles for gene expression because they can be engineered to target expression of biologically active proteins selectively, such as cytokines and growth factors, to mammalian cells [47]. Application of this strategy to the treatment of dogs that have cancer is currently being evaluated. In a recently completed phase I trial, 15 dogs received an intravenous infusion of a TNF-phage construct designed specifically to target tumor vasculature [48]. Pre- and posttreatment tumor biopsies demonstrated that TNF-phage expression was localized to tumor tissue and was not present in adjacent normal tissues. Only 1 dog experienced a dose-limiting hypersensitivity reaction; side effects were not observed in any of the other dogs. A multi-institutional phase II study to assess antitumor efficacy in dogs with a variety of malignancies is currently underway.

Another method designed to increase the efficacy and decrease the toxicity of TNFα therapy is chemical modification with an active ester of monomethoxy–polyethylene glycol (PEG). In mice, PEG-TNFα is much more potent at lower doses than the naive cytokine, because modification increases the plasma half-life and favors accumulation of TNFα within tumor tissues [49–51]. A phase II trial investigating PEG-TNF is currently being conducted in dogs with splenic HSA. After splenectomy, dogs in this study receive PEG-TNF as an intravenous infusion once every 3 weeks for a total of five treatments. Although preliminary results are not yet available, toxicity associated with PEG-TNF has been far less than that seen with administration of unmodified TNFα (D. Thamm, Fort Collins, CO, personal communication, 2007).

TUMOR-SPECIFIC IMMUNOTHERAPY
Unconjugated Monoclonal Antibodies

The use of mAbs specifically to target and treat cancer has been studied for more than 35 years. Since the initial development of hybridoma cell technology by Kohler and Milstein in 1975, mAb therapy has grown to encompass a wide range of malignancies. mAbs are generally designed to target defined tumor-specific antigens or receptors that are frequently overexpressed on malignant cells. mAbs can be used to stimulate antitumor immune responses directly or can be designed to deliver toxins, radionuclide drugs, and cytokines directly to tumor tissue.

Several mAbs are now a part of "standard-of-care" therapy for people with malignancies, such as lymphoma, renal cell cancer, and carcinoma of the breast and colon [52–57]. An example of this is bevacizumab (Avastin), a humanized antibody directed against vascular endothelial growth factor (VEGF), which inhibits tumor angiogenesis. In people, bevacizumab is frequently used in combination with chemotherapy for treatment of renal cell and breast carcinoma and is a part of first-line therapy for metastatic colorectal carcinoma [57,58].

Although designed to inhibit human VEGF, the large degree of sequence homology between canine and human VEGF prompted recent evaluation of bevacizumab's effects on canine tumors [59]. Canine OSA xenografts were established in athymic-nude mice, followed by treatment with high- or low-dose bevacizumab or placebo injection [60]. The mice receiving high-dose therapy demonstrated significantly delayed tumor growth compared with control mice. Although the findings from this study support the continued investigation of bevacizumab in tumor-bearing dogs, repeated administration of a humanized mAb would be expected to elicit the development of antihuman antibodies that could limit the duration of any clinical benefit of bevacizumab in canine patients that have cancer.

Conjugated Monoclonal Antibodies
Immunotoxin-conjugated antibodies
Immunotoxins are mAbs linked to bacterial, plant, or synthetic toxins and are designed to internalize into malignant cells after recognition and binding to a defined tumor-associated antigen. Once internalized, the toxin is released from the antibody and induces cell death by means of several mechanisms, such as inhibition of protein synthesis.

The best studied immunotoxin in veterinary oncology is BR96 sFv-PE40. BR96 is a mouse mAb that recognizes a carbohydrate antigen (Lewis^y [Le^y]) expressed by a wide variety of solid tumors in mice and human beings [61]. BR96, conjugated to an exotoxin derived from *Pseudomonas*, binds efficiently to human breast and lung carcinoma xenografts in rodents and triggers tumor apoptosis [62,63]. To determine whether BR96 sFv-PE40 is useful in the treatment of dogs that have carcinoma, tumor tissue samples were obtained from client-owned dogs and screened for expression of the Le^y antigen [64]. Twenty-two of 61 carcinomas, including samples obtained from dogs with mammary, prostate, lung, and rectal carcinoma, were found to be positive for the antigen. Twelve of these dogs were then entered into a phase I/II clinical trial to assess the immunotoxin's safety and efficacy. The dogs received twice-weekly infusions of BR96 sFv-PE40 at a dose of 4 to 12 mg/m^2. The primary toxicities were fever and vomiting, both of which resolved within 24 hours. Partial remission or stable disease was achieved in 6 of the 12 dogs; however, unfortunately, anti-immunotoxin antibodies developed in 9 dogs after two to five infusions. It is hoped that combination of BR96 sFv-PE40 with chemotherapeutic agents might decrease the tendency for antibody development to occur; this approach is to be explored in future clinical trials.

Radionuclide-conjugated antibodies
Radiolabeled mAbs deliver radioisotopes to tumor tissue while sparing normal organs and tissues. Because the energy released by radiolabeled mAbs penetrates more effectively into bulky solid tumors than unconjugated antibodies are able to do, the radionuclide antibodies are attractive for their potential use in patients with large tumor burdens.

The primary application of the radionuclide-conjugated antibodies in veterinary oncology is in tumor imaging. For example, a ^{125}Iodine (I)-labeled antibody directed against Met, a tyrosine kinase receptor that is overexpressed in a variety of malignancies, was recently evaluated in canine prostatic carcinoma [65]. Using prostatic carcinoma tumor xenografts established in mice as a model, the investigators found that intravenous administration of the ^{125}I-Met antibody led to gradual mAb uptake within tumor tissue, peaking at 1 day after injection and persisting for at least 5 days. This technique permitted clear delineation of normal tissue from tumor tissue and suggested that the radiolabeled antibody might be a useful immunotherapeutic agent because of its long persistence within tumor tissue.

A separate study examined the ability of an ^{111}Indium (In)-labeled mAb, reactive with canine prostatic carcinoma, to target tumor tissue in a dog with advanced metastatic disease [66]. Pretreatment ultrasonography in this patient had revealed tumor metastasis to a single sublumbar lymph node. Nuclear imaging after administration of the radiolabeled mAb revealed ^{111}In uptake within multiple sublumbar lymph nodes and the left adrenal gland, however. The dog was euthanized a short time later, and a necropsy confirmed the more widespread metastatic disease detected by nuclear imaging. Future studies are likely to assess targeted antitumor effects in addition to the imaging capabilities of radionuclide-conjugated mAbs.

CHALLENGES FOR THE FUTURE

In this article, the author has reviewed the major types of immunotherapy (with the exception of tumor vaccines, which are discussed elsewhere in this issue) under investigation in preclinical studies or currently being evaluated in clinical trials for dogs and cats with cancer. Ideally, immunotherapy is designed to engage the immune system in the recognition and attack of malignant cells with the goal of controlling, or even preventing, the growth of a primary tumor and providing protection against the development of metastatic disease. Strategies to achieve this goal include stimulation of the immune system as a whole (the biologic response modifiers and cytokines); selective activation of tumor-specific lymphocytes (tumor vaccines); targeted delivery of antibodies, toxins, or radioisotopes to tumor tissue (tumor-specific immunotherapy).

Some of the immunotherapeutics discussed in this section cause significant toxicity when administered systemically, especially when given in high doses. Others seem to be most useful when used along with conventional cytotoxic chemotherapy agents. These factors are among the reasons for the current trend toward combination of immunotherapy with traditional anticancer treatments, such as surgery, radiation therapy, and chemotherapy. Although this trend opens up a whole new world of possibilities in treating cancer, it also presents several obstacles and challenges. For example, determination of appropriate clinical and biologic end points is now one of the biggest hurdles in immunotherapy trial design. Chemotherapy agents typically induce rapid tumor cell death that is detectable within a few days. The clinical response to an immunotherapy agent, however, may depend on the development of an adaptive immune response that can take several months or more to appear. Therefore, trials must be planned in such a way as to allow adequate time for the appropriate response to develop and to take into account the possible effects of other therapies.

Another potential problem in determining treatment outcome is the observation of "mixed responses" in clinical trials involving patients with metastatic disease. This phenomenon is characterized by the differential response to therapy within different tissues of the same patient. Because of this problem, a new set of monitoring criteria was recently proposed by the National Cancer Institute. Called RECIST (response evaluation criteria in solid tumors), an objective clinical response is now defined as a 30% reduction in the sum of the maximum diameters of lesions and the appearance of no new or progressive lesions [67].

Despite challenges like these, immunotherapy offers much promise in improving our present ability to control cancer. The veterinary profession, in particular, should be critically important in moving the ideas of basic research into the clinic because of the tremendous value of companion animals as translational models. In general, dogs and cats are much more likely to predict treatment response and toxicity in people than are mouse models of cancer. Many tumors, such as OSA, melanoma, and non-Hodgkin's lymphoma, exhibit markedly similar behavior between companion animals and human beings. We, as veterinarians, therefore have an unparalleled opportunity to develop and evaluate therapies that can potentially benefit human and veterinary species.

References

[1] Coley W. The treatment of inoperable sarcoma by bacterial toxins (the mixed toxins of Streptococcus erysipelas and the Bacillus prodigiosus). Proceedings of the Royal Society of Medicine (Surgical Section) 1909;3(1):1–48.
[2] McCarthy EF. The toxins of William B. Coley and the treatment of bone and soft-tissue sarcomas. Iowa Orthop J 2006;26:154–8.
[3] Alexandroff AB, Jackson AM, O'Donnell MA, et al. BCG immunotherapy of bladder cancer: 20 years on. Lancet 1999;353(9165):1689–94.
[4] van der Meijden AP. Non-specific immunotherapy with bacille Calmette-Guerin (BCG). Clin Exp Immunol 2001;123(2):179–80.
[5] Chen X, O'Donnell MA, Luo Y. Dose-dependent synergy of Th1-stimulating cytokines on bacille Calmette-Guerin-induced interferon-gamma production by human mononuclear cells. Clin Exp Immunol 2007;149(1):178–85.
[6] Luo Y, Yamada H, Chen X, et al. Recombinant Mycobacterium bovis bacillus Calmette-Guerin (BCG) expressing mouse IL-18 augments Th1 immunity and macrophage cytotoxicity. Clin Exp Immunol 2004;137(1):24–34.
[7] Knapp DW, Jacobs RM. Naturally-occurring canine transitional cell carcinoma of the urinary bladder: a relevant model of human invasive bladder cancer. Urol Oncol 2000; 5:47–59.
[8] van der Meijden AP, Steerenberg PA, de Jong WH, et al. The effects of intravesical and intradermal application of a new B.C.G. on the dog bladder. Urol Res 1986;14(4):207–10.
[9] Klein WR, Rutten VP, Steerenberg PA, et al. The present status of BCG treatment in the veterinary practice. In Vivo 1991;5(6):605–8.
[10] Rutten VP, Klein WR, De Jong WA, et al. Immunotherapy of bovine ocular squamous cell carcinoma by repeated intralesional injections of live bacillus Calmette-Guerin (BCG) or BCG cell walls. Cancer Immunol Immunother 1991;34(3):186–90.

[11] Henry C. Clinical comparison of LDI-100, a preparation containing human chorionic gonadotropin and bacillus Calmette-Guerin, to single-agent vinblastine for the treatment of canine mast cell tumors. Paper presented at: Veterinary Cancer Society Annual Conference. Pine Mountain (GA), October 19–22, 2006.

[12] Knapp D. Antitumor activity of mycobacterial cell wall-DNA complex (MCC) against canine urinary bladder transitional cell carcinoma cells. Paper presented at: Veterinary Cancer Society Annual Conference Proceedings. Kansas City (MO), November 3–6, 2004.

[13] Filion MC, Phillips NC. Therapeutic potential of mycobacterial cell wall-DNA complexes. Expert Opin Investig Drugs 2001;10(12):2157–65.

[14] Filion MC, Filion B, Phillips NC. Effects of mycobacterial cell wall-DNA complexes (MCC), alendronate and pamidronate on canine osteosarcoma cell lines. Paper presented at: Veterinary Cancer Society Annual Conference. Kansas City (MO), November 3–6, 2004.

[15] Nardin A, Lefebvre ML, Labroquere K, et al. Liposomal muramyl tripeptide phosphatidylethanolamine: targeting and activating macrophages for adjuvant treatment of osteosarcoma. Curr Cancer Drug Targets 2006;6(2):123–33.

[16] Fox LE, MacEwen EG, Kurzman ID, et al. Liposome-encapsulated muramyl tripeptide phosphatidylethanolamine for the treatment of feline mammary adenocarcinoma—a multicenter randomized double-blind study. Cancer Biother 1995;10(2):125–30.

[17] Vail DM, MacEwen EG, Kurzman ID, et al. Liposome-encapsulated muramyl tripeptide phosphatidylethanolamine adjuvant immunotherapy for splenic hemangiosarcoma in the dog: a randomized multi-institutional clinical trial. Clin Cancer Res 1995;1(10):1165–70.

[18] Kurzman ID, MacEwen EG, Rosenthal RC, et al. Adjuvant therapy for osteosarcoma in dogs: results of randomized clinical trials using combined liposome-encapsulated muramyl tripeptide and cisplatin. Clin Cancer Res 1995;1(12):1595–601.

[19] MacEwen EG, Rosenthal RC. Combined liposome-encapsulated muramyl tripeptide and cisplatin in dogs with osteosarcoma. In: Novak JFMJ, editor. Frontiers of osteosarcoma research. Toronto: Hogrefe and Huber; 1993. p. 117–9.

[20] MacEwen EG, Kurzman ID, Vail DM, et al. Adjuvant therapy for melanoma in dogs: results of randomized clinical trials using surgery, liposome-encapsulated muramyl tripeptide, and granulocyte macrophage colony-stimulating factor. Clin Cancer Res 1999;5(12):4249–58.

[21] Teske E, Rutteman GR, vd Ingh TS, et al. Liposome-encapsulated muramyl tripeptide phosphatidylethanolamine (L-MTP-PE): a randomized clinical trial in dogs with mammary carcinoma. Anticancer Res 1998;18(2A):1015–9.

[22] Dow SW, Fradkin LG, Liggitt DH, et al. Lipid-DNA complexes induce potent activation of innate immune responses and antitumor activity when administered intravenously. J Immunol 1999;163(3):1552–61.

[23] Gursel I, Gursel M, Ishii KJ, et al. Sterically stabilized cationic liposomes improve the uptake and immunostimulatory activity of CpG oligonucleotides. J Immunol 2001;167(6):3324–8.

[24] U'Ren L, Kedl R, Dow S. Vaccination with liposome-DNA complexes elicits enhanced antitumor immunity. Cancer Gene Ther 2006;13(11):1033–44.

[25] Whitmore M, Li S, Huang L. LPD lipopolyplex initiates a potent cytokine response and inhibits tumor growth. Gene Ther 1999;6(11):1867–75.

[26] Whitmore MM, Li S, Falo L Jr, et al. Systemic administration of LPD prepared with CpG oligonucleotides inhibits the growth of established pulmonary metastases by stimulating innate and acquired antitumor immune responses. Cancer Immunol Immunother 2001;50(10):503–14.

[27] U'Ren L, Biller B, Elmslie R, Rose B, et al. Evaluation of an allogeneic tumor vaccine in dogs with oral melanoma. Paper presented at: Veterinary Cancer Society Annual Conference. Kansas City (MO), November 3–6, 2004.

[28] U'Ren LW, Biller BJ, Elmslie RE, et al. Evaluation of a novel tumor vaccine in dogs with hemangiosarcoma. J Vet Intern Med 2007;21(1):113–20.

[29] Anwer K, Kao G, Proctor B, et al. Optimization of cationic lipid/DNA complexes for systemic gene transfer to tumor lesions. J Drug Target 2000;8(2):125–35.
[30] Dow S, Elmslie R, Kurzman I, et al. Phase I study of liposome-DNA complexes encoding the interleukin-2 gene in dogs with osteosarcoma lung metastases. Hum Gene Ther 2005;16(8):937–46.
[31] Kamstock D, Guth A, Elmslie R, et al. Liposome-DNA complexes infused intravenously inhibit tumor angiogenesis and elicit antitumor activity in dogs with soft tissue sarcoma. Cancer Gene Ther 2006;13(3):306–17.
[32] Chiocca EA. Oncolytic viruses. Nat Rev Cancer 2002;2(12):938–50.
[33] Suter SE, Chein MB, von Messling V, et al. In vitro canine distemper virus infection of canine lymphoid cells: a prelude to oncolytic therapy for lymphoma. Clin Cancer Res 2005;11(4):1579–87.
[34] Candolfi M, Kroeger KM, Pluhar GE, et al. Adenoviral-mediated gene transfer into the canine brain in vivo. Neurosurgery 2007;60(1):167–77 [discussion: 178].
[35] Le LP, Rivera AA, Glasgow JN, et al. Infectivity enhancement for adenoviral transduction of canine osteosarcoma cells. Gene Ther 2006;13(5):389–99.
[36] Le LP, Li J, Ternovoi VV, et al. Fluorescently tagged canine adenovirus via modification with protein IX-enhanced green fluorescent protein. J Gen Virol 2005;86(Pt 12):3201–8.
[37] Thompson JA, Peace DJ, Klarnet JP, et al. Eradication of disseminated murine leukemia by treatment with high-dose interleukin 2. J Immunol 1986;137(11):3675–80.
[38] Khanna C, Anderson PM, Hasz DE, et al. Interleukin-2 liposome inhalation therapy is safe and effective for dogs with spontaneous pulmonary metastases. Cancer 1997;79(7):1409–21.
[39] Esteban-Gonzalez E, Carballido J, Navas V, et al. Retrospective review in patients with pulmonary metastases of renal cell carcinoma receiving inhaled recombinant interleukin-2. Anticancer Drugs 2007;18(3):291–6.
[40] Buttner M, Belke-Louis G, Rziha HJ, et al. Detection, cDNA cloning and sequencing of canine interleukin 12. Cytokine 1998;10(4):241–8.
[41] Okano F, Satoh M, Yamada K. Cloning and expression of the cDNA for canine interleukin-12. J Interferon Cytokine Res 1997;17(11):713–8.
[42] Phillips BS, Padilla ML, Dickerson EB, et al. Immunostimulatory effects of human recombinant interleukin-12 on peripheral blood mononuclear cells from normal dogs. Vet Immunol Immunopathol 1999;70(3–4):189–201.
[43] Akhtar N, Padilla ML, Dickerson EB, et al. Interleukin-12 inhibits tumor growth in a novel angiogenesis canine hemangiosarcoma xenograft model. Neoplasia 2004;6(2):106–16.
[44] Siddiqui F, Li CY, Larue SM, et al. A phase I trial of hyperthermia-induced interleukin-12 gene therapy in spontaneously arising feline soft tissue sarcomas. Mol Cancer Ther 2007;6(1):380–9.
[45] Ruegg C, Yilmaz A, Bieler G, et al. Evidence for the involvement of endothelial cell integrin alphaVbeta3 in the disruption of the tumor vasculature induced by TNF and IFN-gamma. Nat Med 1998;4(4):408–14.
[46] Schweigerer L, Malerstein B, Gospodarowicz D. Tumor necrosis factor inhibits the proliferation of cultured capillary endothelial cells. Biochem Biophys Res Commun 1987;143(3):997–1004.
[47] Larocca D, Kassner PD, Witte A, et al. Gene transfer to mammalian cells using genetically targeted filamentous bacteriophage. FASEB J 1999;13(6):727–34.
[48] Paoloni M. Evaluation of RGD targeted delivery of phage expressing TNF-alpha to tumor bearing dogs: the inaugural trial of the Comparative Oncology Trials Consortium. Paper presented at: Veterinary Cancer Society Annual Conference. Pine Mountain (GA), October 19–22, 2006.
[49] Tsunoda S, Ishikawa T, Yamamoto Y, et al. Enhanced antitumor potency of polyethylene glycosylated tumor necrosis factor-alpha: a novel polymer-conjugation technique with a reversible amino-protective reagent. J Pharmacol Exp Ther 1999;290(1):368–72.

[50] Tsutsumi Y, Kihira T, Tsunoda S, et al. Molecular design of hybrid tumor necrosis factor-alpha III: polyethylene glycol-modified tumor necrosis factor-alpha has markedly enhanced antitumor potency due to longer plasma half-life and higher tumor accumulation. J Pharmacol Exp Ther 1996;278(3):1006–11.

[51] Tsutsumi Y, Kihira T, Yamamoto S, et al. Chemical modification of natural human tumor necrosis factor-alpha with polyethylene glycol increases its anti-tumor potency. Jpn J Cancer Res 1994;85(1):9–12.

[52] Fernando NH, Hurwitz HI. Targeted therapy of colorectal cancer: clinical experience with bevacizumab. Oncologist 2004;9(Suppl 1):11–8.

[53] McLaughlin P, White CA, Grillo-Lopez AJ, et al. Clinical status and optimal use of rituximab for B-cell lymphomas. Oncology 1998;12(12):1763–9 [discussion: 1769–70, 1775–67].

[54] Rugo HS. Bevacizumab in the treatment of breast cancer: rationale and current data. Oncologist 2004;9(Suppl 1):43–9.

[55] Slamon DJ, Leyland-Jones B, Shak S, et al. Use of chemotherapy plus a monoclonal antibody against HER2 for metastatic breast cancer that overexpresses HER2. N Engl J Med. 15 2001;344(11):783–92.

[56] Stern M, Herrmann R. Overview of monoclonal antibodies in cancer therapy: present and promise. Crit Rev Oncol Hematol 2005;54(1):11–29.

[57] Yang JC, Haworth L, Sherry RM, et al. A randomized trial of bevacizumab, an anti-vascular endothelial growth factor antibody, for metastatic renal cancer. N Engl J Med 2003;349(5): 427–34.

[58] Hurwitz H, Fehrenbacher L, Novotny W, et al. Bevacizumab plus irinotecan, fluorouracil, and leucovorin for metastatic colorectal cancer. N Engl J Med 2004;350(23):2335–42.

[59] Scheidegger P, Weiglhofer W, Suarez S, et al. Vascular endothelial growth factor (VEGF) and its receptors in tumor-bearing dogs. Biol Chem 1999;380(12):1449–54.

[60] Farese J. Avastin-bevacizumab delays growth of xenografted canine osteosarcoma in a murine model. Paper presented at: Veterinary Cancer Society Annual Conference. Pine Mountain (GA), October 19–22, 2006.

[61] Hellstrom I, Garrigues HJ, Garrigues U, et al. Highly tumor-reactive, internalizing, mouse monoclonal antibodies to Le(y)-related cell surface antigens. Cancer Res 1990;50(7): 2183–90.

[62] Friedman PN, Chace DF, Trail PA, et al. Antitumor activity of the single-chain immunotoxin BR96 sFv-PE40 against established breast and lung tumor xenografts. J Immunol 1993;150(7):3054–61.

[63] Siegall CB, Chace D, Mixan B, et al. In vitro and in vivo characterization of BR96 sFv-PE40. A single-chain immunotoxin fusion protein that cures human breast carcinoma xenografts in athymic mice and rats. J Immunol 1994;152(5):2377–84.

[64] Henry CJ, Buss MS, Hellstrom I, et al. Clinical evaluation of BR96 sFv-PE40 immunotoxin therapy in canine models of spontaneously occurring invasive carcinoma. Clin Cancer Res 2005;11(2 Pt 1):751–5.

[65] Hay RV, Cao B, Skinner RS, et al. Nuclear imaging of Met-expressing human and canine cancer xenografts with radiolabeled monoclonal antibodies (MetSeek). Clin Cancer Res 2005;11(19 Pt 2):7064s–9s.

[66] Lewis M. Antibody pretargeting for molecular imaging of canine metastatic prostate cancer. Paper presented at: Veterinary Cancer Society Annual Conference. Huntington Beach (CA), October 20–23, 2005.

[67] Rosenberg SA, Yang JC, Restifo NP. Cancer immunotherapy: moving beyond current vaccines. Nat Med 2004;10(9):909–15.

Intensity-Modulated Radiation Therapy and Helical Tomotherapy: Its Origin, Benefits, and Potential Applications in Veterinary Medicine

Jessica A. Lawrence, DVM[a], Lisa J. Forrest, VMD[b],*

[a]Department of Medical Sciences, University of Wisconsin-Madison, 2015 Linden Drive, Madison, WI 53706, USA
[b]Department of Surgical Sciences, University of Wisconsin-Madison, 2015 Linden Drive, Madison, WI 53706, USA

Radiation dose delivered to a patient affects tumor-containing tissue as well as normal tissues. The biologic effect of radiation on these tissues depends on several factors, including the magnitude of the delivered dose, the fractionation scheme, and the sensitivity of the tissue [1–3]. The goal in radiation oncology is to attain a high degree of tumor control with minimal deleterious effects, but a compromise between tumor control and normal tissue side effects is more often realistically achievable. Conformal radiation therapy has been proposed as a means to improve the efficacy of radiation therapy by more appropriately collimating the treatment field to the target tumor volume [4]. Tomotherapy is an advanced form of conformal intensity-modulated radiation therapy (IMRT) that also uses image verification to deliver radiation to the desired target precisely. One reason why radiation therapy fails to provide local tumor control is that a lethal dose of radiation cannot be delivered to the target tumor volume without severely injuring adjacent normal tissue. The delivery of targeted radiation represents an opportunity for radiation oncologists to escalate dose to the tumor volume while minimizing dose to surrounding tissues. This idea of targeted therapy poses several potential benefits for human and veterinary patients not only in terms of improved control of malignancies but to limit detrimental effects on quality of life.

THREE-DIMENSIONAL CONFORMAL RADIATION THERAPY

Before appreciating tomotherapy and its applications, an understanding of conformal and intensity-modulated techniques is useful. The rationale behind

---

This work was supported by National Cancer Institute grant 1PO1 CA88960.

*Corresponding author. E-mail address: forrestl@svm.vetmed.wisc.edu (L.J. Forrest).

three-dimensional (3D) conformal radiation therapy is to maximize the difference between radiation dose delivered to the tumor versus the surrounding normal tissue. 3D conformal radiation therapy was developed in the 1980s and significantly improved the therapeutic ratio [3,5]. Conformal radiation allows an increase in dose to the tumor volume by narrowing the radiation field to fit the shape of the tumor volume, and in doing so, it attempts to minimize dose to surrounding normal tissue [4,6]. Delivery of 3D conformal radiation treatments uses 3D image visualization and treatment planning tools to conform isodose distributions to target volumes while excluding as much normal tissue as possible [6]. Isodose distributions provide visualization of the dose delivered to different points within the target medium and surrounding the target. The goal in radiation treatment planning is to create a uniform dose distribution (isodose) within the tumor volume to avoid over- and underdosage. In fact, based on this technology, 3D conformal radiation therapy has thus far provided a means for safe escalation of target dose to a significant number of patients, which should translate into improved local tumor control and quality of life [7–9].

Treatment planning is entirely image based, and patient anatomy is evaluated by CT. Tumor volumes and critical structures are outlined using contouring tools and can be evaluated three dimensionally. The volume of tumor and normal tissue that is irradiated depends on several factors [5,10]. The gross tumor volume (GTV) refers to the volume of tissue that is visibly abnormal by means of imaging methods. A specific margin is added to this GTV to create a clinical tumor volume (CTV) to account for the presence of microscopic disease. A second margin of tissue is added to the CTV to create a planning target volume (PTV) to account for daily setup variability and organ motion. Because of the fact that patients are not set up identically for each treatment, the PTV is generally considered the target volume. Conventional forward planning is used, implying that the planner enters and adjusts radiation beams and beam modifiers to formulate an optimal dose distribution for a particular patient [6,10]. Generally, several modified beams are oriented in different directions to conform the volume irradiated to an irregular and appropriate shape. Multileaf collimators (MLCs) are used in some linear accelerators to shape the radiation beam. MLCs consist of anywhere from 52 to 120 metal leaves that slide into place to create a desired field shape and are ideal for complex and irregular treatment volumes.

INTENSITY-MODULATED RADIATION THERAPY AND CONFORMAL AVOIDANCE

IMRT and 3D conformal radiation therapy allow for the possibility to optimize dose delivery to complex target volumes, further allowing targeted treatment [11–13]. Despite its name, however, 3D conformal radiation therapy does not conform well to a particular shape unless a large number of beams are used and the target has a relatively simple shape [14]. For complex shapes, such as a tumor that wraps around a spinal cord, there is no acceptable 3D conformal plan that can be designed [14]. Intensity modulation techniques take 3D conformal radiation therapy one step further by allowing modification of intensity distribution within a treatment beam to maximize the dose to the target volume further while minimizing the dose to critical structures [5,6]. IMRT employs the use of MLCs to create desired treatment field shapes along with intensity alterations for each field [5,6]. The metal leaves of the MLC are arranged to slide into place to create a desired field shape before treatment (segmental IMRT) or during treatment (dynamic IMRT) [14]. The linear accelerator's computer system controls the MLC leaves to alter the shape and duration of the beams during treatment delivery. Similar to 3D conformal radiation therapy, IMRT is most often delivered by using multiple beam directions with the utilization of several small collimated fields, often with several subfields per beam direction [14]. A larger number of treatment beams are required for IMRT, and the treatment plans tend to take longer to devise than with conventional conformal treatment planning. Although forward treatment planning can be done if the target is relatively simple; in general, IMRT requires the use of inverse treatment planning programs, however. In this case, the planner defines the desired dose to the target tissues and the number of beams and beam directions, but the computer program devises the optimal intensity distribution for each beam that results in the best approximation to the desired dose distribution within the planner's constraints [14]. The advent of numerous small radiation fields, as opposed to conventional three- or four-field arrangements, inherently increases inaccuracies associated with radiation delivery, because there is a steeper dose gradient for IMRT plans compared with conventional 3D conformal plans [5,14]. IMRT plans devised and calculated for different tumors, including those in the nasopharynx, prostate, liver, lung, and paraspinal regions, have yielded significantly better dose distributions compared with plans made with 3D conformal radiation therapy systems [14–18]. In theory, this represents a method of improving tumor control while reducing toxicity to normal structures, provided the radiation oncologist can control and verify the dose delivery to the targeted tumor volume.

CONFORMAL AVOIDANCE

Complementary to the idea of conformal radiation therapy, whether by conventional means or by IMRT, is the idea of conformal avoidance [5,19]. Rather than trying to map the precise area to be treated, critical structures can be mapped out so that radiation to those areas is avoided [5,19]. Conformal avoidance is essentially an "everything but" treatment plan, and as such, there tends to be a rapid decrease in radiation dose near sensitive structures [5]. This concept again implies that the patient must be accurately positioned to maintain the high dose gradient in the proper location. This is likely the major criticism of conventional IMRT in that the relative position and shape of the tumor and critical organs are not certain at each treatment setup [20]. A relatively large margin (PTV) is required during dose delivery to avoid a geographic miss, and because margins around the tumor volume shrink with conformal therapy, it is extremely important to ensure appropriate patient and beam positioning.

HUMAN HEAD AND NECK CANCER AND CONFORMAL AVOIDANCE

Probably the most popular example of clinical applications of conformal avoidance involves the sparing of the major salivary glands during head and neck radiation therapy. Human patients undergoing head and neck radiation commonly experience significant local toxicity to the parotid salivary glands, and xerostomia represents a chronic and ongoing problem. Xerostomia is associated with taste impairment, difficulty in chewing and swallowing, increased incidence of dental caries and oral candidiasis, and difficulty in speaking. This has a major impact on patient quality-of-life deterioration and satisfaction after radiation therapy. Temporary symptomatic relief is afforded by the use of moistening agents and saliva substitutes in patients who have minimal salivary gland function. Oral pilocarpine may increase salivary flow and ameliorate symptoms of xerostomia in patients who have some residual salivary gland function, but this has not been corroborated by several studies [21–23]. This emphasizes the importance of sparing some salivary gland tissue during radiation therapy, because medical management may be beneficial even if the entire gland cannot be spared [24]. Amifostine, a thiol-containing chemotherapy and radiation protector, is currently approved for xerostomia prevention in the postoperative head and neck cancer therapy setting [25,26]. The initial phase III trial demonstrated a reduced incidence of clinically significant xerostomia in patients receiving radiotherapy treated with amifostine (34%) compared with those not receiving amifostine (57%) [25]. In a 2-year follow up study, amifostine reduced the severity and duration of xerostomia after treatment and did not compromise locoregional control rates, progression-free survival, or overall survival [26]. Although these results showed promise, the overall benefit of using amifostine remains low and further techniques to reduce patient discomfort and chronic damage are needed.

There are several early studies indicating that patients treated with IMRT experience significantly more parotid gland sparing compared with those treated with conventional 3D radiation therapy [27–31]. In one study evaluating a small number of patients (N = 23) receiving head and neck radiation therapy by means of inverse-planned intensity-modulated delivery, oral health-related issues were highly preserved within the initial 12 months after therapy [29]. Additionally, the number of patients reporting xerostomia-related quality-of-life issues was not significantly different from baseline, indicating reasonable preservation of salivary function [29]. In a separate evaluation of quality-of-life issues and xerostomia, patients treated with IMRT for head and neck cancer experienced significant benefit 6 months and longer after treatment compared with patients treated with 3D conformal radiation therapy [31]. These studies are ongoing as IMRT is more widely used in a variety of academic and private facilities.

Whereas head and neck radiation therapy impairs normal salivary gland function in people, a comparable toxicity in veterinary patients is the development of ocular toxicity in dogs with nasal tumors treated with radiation therapy. Nasal tumors in the dog comprise approximately 1% to 2% of all neoplasms in this species [32,33]. Tumors can arise from a multitude of tissues, although carcinomas and sarcomas are the first and second most commonly diagnosed nasal tumors, respectively. Radiation therapy is considered to be the most effective means of achieving local tumor control, although tumor recurrence occurs in most cases and median survival times range from approximately 8 to 19.7 months [34–38]. Improvement in survival has been described in a small number of dogs treated with radiation therapy followed by exenteration of the nasal cavity in those cases with residual disease, but larger studies need to corroborate this finding [38]. Regardless of the addition of surgery or not, radiation therapy can induce several side effects that can affect patient and owner quality of life. Acute side effects vary from mild to severe depending on the prescribed protocol, and effects consist of oral mucositis, halitosis, skin erythema and marked desquamation, and conjunctivitis. Although acute side effects typically heal within several weeks of discontinuation of radiation therapy, a large proportion of dogs treated experience late toxicity in the form of ocular toxicity. Keratoconjunctivitis sicca (KCS), corneal ulceration and secondary uveitis, chronic conjunctivitis, and cataract formation are potential consequences of radiation if the eyes receive doses greater than approximately 40 Gy [39]. Cataract formation and conjunctivitis can be managed fairly successfully, but persistent and poorly controlled KCS and uveitis can be extremely painful and difficult to treat in some cases without enucleation. Improvement in targeted dose delivery using intensity-modulated or conformal avoidance techniques would likely confer significant benefit to veterinary patients undergoing head and neck irradiation. Durable local tumor control continues to be a challenge in canine nasal tumors, and dose escalation may represent an ideal method to improve duration of control while minimizing the occurrence of late ocular effects.

IMAGE-GUIDED RADIATION THERAPY AND HELICAL TOMOTHERAPY

Image-guided radiation therapy seeks to remove uncertainties associated with anatomic positioning at each treatment by acquiring images of the patient immediately before beam delivery on the treatment machine [5,19,20]. The goal of 3D image-guided radiation therapy systems is to reduce the uncertainties associated with microscopic disease, daily patient setup, and interfraction organ motion [5]. Imaging modalities that may prove helpful include CT, MRI, ultrasound, and positron emission tomography (PET)/CT among others. These modalities, with the exception of PET/CT capabilities, are currently widely available and used by a significant number of veterinary practitioners and radiation oncologists. The challenge has been learning to combine image acquisition with treatment delivery in a consistent and reliable manner such that dose delivery to patients coincides with prescribed dose.

Combining imaging with treatment has been a focus of researchers, and helical tomotherapy represents the first clinically useful image-guided, precise, and conformal radiation therapy delivery technique [5,19,40,41]. The helical tomotherapy unit represents the fusion of a linear accelerator with a helical CT scanner and is a dedicated image-guided IMRT system [5]. The linear accelerator sits on a CT ring gantry and has a binary MLC that modulates each beam during treatment to provide rotational and targeted IMRT [5]. Patients are continuously moved (translated) through the ring gantry as the linear accelerator rotates, resulting in a helical course around the patient. Radiation beam delivery is similar to spiral CT and uses similar slip rings for power and data acquisition. The ring gantry provides a fixed and precise structure by which to obtain tomographic verification of the patient setup and dose of radiation delivered. Helical tomotherapy uses a system similar to the NOMOS Peacock system (NOMOS, Corp., Sewickley, Pennsylvania), which employs a fan beam delivered by means of an arcing gantry equipped with an MLC [19,42]. Helical tomotherapy allows for continuous delivery of radiation beams over 360°, however, because the fan beam is attached to a standard C-arm linear accelerator [19]. The obvious advantage of helical tomotherapy over other IMRT systems is the ability for verification of radiation delivery by means of tomographic imaging. Another advantage of helical tomotherapy is that the treatment beam is delivered as a continuous helix, which allows minimization of treatment time and reduction in significant high or low dose deposition in overlap or gap fields, respectively [19,42].

Tomographic images are obtained using the helical tomotherapy unit itself. Patients are positioned on the treatment table in preparation for radiation therapy with careful positioning and alignment. Megavoltage CT (MVCT) images are obtained immediately before treatment that provide sufficient detail for verification and registration of the patient [5,40,42]. Images acquired with the helical tomotherapy unit are typically obtained at radiation doses of approximately 2 cGy, similar to that of diagnostic CT imaging, so that patients are not exposed to excessive doses before treatment [40,42,43]. Researchers at the University of Wisconsin-Madison are currently evaluating cone-beam kilovoltage CT (kVCT) technology and comparing it with helical tomotherapy MVCT capabilities, and continuing work may further reduce the dose to patients and allow improved image quality [42].

Patients are initially scanned for approximately 90 to 180 seconds depending on the slice thickness selected. During the scanning process, the initial treatment planning kVCT axial images can be visualized directly against the current day's MVCT images. Patient positioning can be roughly evaluated, but the tomotherapy software directly fuses the MVCT scan with the original planning kVCT scan (Fig. 1). Fusion is done quickly, first by automated methods, and is ultimately fine-tuned manually [5,40]. Setup correction includes translational (lateral, longitudinal, and vertical shifts) and rotational

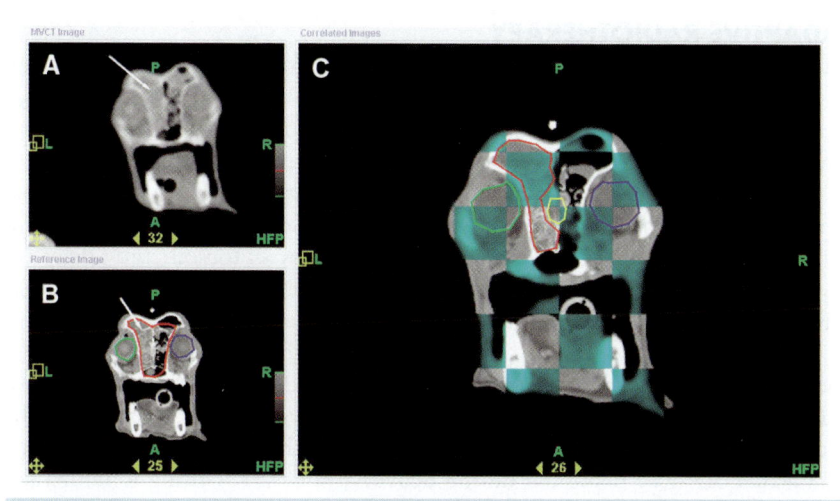

Fig. 1. MVCT (A), kVCT (B), and aligned (C, correlated) images of the nasal cavity of a dog with a nasopharyngeal tumor at the level of the eyes. Note the tumor filling the left nasal cavity and extending to the right (*white arrows*). In images B and C, the contours from left to right are left eye (*green*), nasal cavity tumor (*red*), rostral brain (*C, yellow*), and right eye (*blue*). On the aligned (C, correlated) image, the teal checkerboard regions represent the MVCT image superimposed over the kVCT image. (*From* Forrest LJ, Mackie TR, Ruchala K, et al. The utility of megavoltage computed tomography images from a helical tomotherapy system for setup verification purposes. Int J Radiat Oncol Biol Phys 2004;60(5):1641; with permission.)

(yaw, pitch, and roll) information for accurately correcting the patient position before treatment [5]. All translational and roll adjustments can be made without moving the patient, because the tomotherapy unit software transfers most of these transformations directly to the couch. Lateral changes are done manually by moving the couch. Yaw and pitch present a more complicated approach to adjustment and must be manually adjusted. If only minor adjustment is required and the oncologist is satisfied, treatment can be instituted. If a major adjustment has been made manually, a repeat MVCT scan is often obtained to ensure that the patient is in the correct position for treatment. The use of deep vacuum-formable mattresses and localizing tools helps to minimize pitch and yaw on daily setups. Once the patient has been precisely positioned to match the original (planned) position, the tomotherapy beam is turned on and the treatment is initialized. The overall treatment time is longer than with conventional linear accelerators and cobalt teletherapy units, with the setup verification taking approximately 5 minutes in total and treatment delivery times ranging from 5 to 7 minutes [40]. Because radiation is delivered continuously in a helical manner with the couch moving forward into the bore of the gantry, however, treatment times are shorter than conventional IMRT plans. Veterinary patients are anesthetized for each treatment and are typically under anesthesia for approximately 20 to 25 minutes.

ADAPTIVE RADIOTHERAPY

Adaptive radiotherapy is a concept that refers to the process of applying feedback directly to the image-guided radiotherapy process [5,44]. This allows the radiation oncologist to verify and adjust the therapeutic plan as needed throughout the course of a patient's treatment. Adaptive radiotherapy involves a closed-circuit loop consisting of optimized CT-based planning for conformal therapy and conformal avoidance therapy, processes for precise pretreatment evaluation of patient positioning, improved accuracy of tomotherapy delivery, and posttreatment dosimetry to evaluate and enable adaptive therapy further (Fig. 2) [42].

Radiation delivery cannot normally be rapidly assessed and adjusted, because dosimetry results obtained from thermoluminescent dosimeters (TLDs) or other verification methods require several days to process. The development of dose reconstruction tools offers the capability to determine the actual 3D dose deposited during delivery, however. During tomotherapy treatment, exit detectors on the machine compute the incident energy fluence from the MLC while a detailed 3D representation of the patient is being obtained [42]. The integrated CT within the tomotherapy unit provides scatter characteristics for each projection and path length, and detector-to-patient distances can be calculated directly from the MVCT images [42]. The treatment dose distribution is ultimately computed using a convolution/superposition algorithm, which has excellent accuracy [42,45]. This effectively results in the generation of a daily pictorial dose record and can be directly compared with the planned dose distribution for the patient [42]. Comparative information could be assessed on a daily basis or after several fractions have been administered. Potential advantages include recognition of setup error because of changes in tumor geometry or organ movements such that adjustments could be made for the remaining fractions to account for decreased or increased dose to the tumor volume or critical organs. A challenge that remains

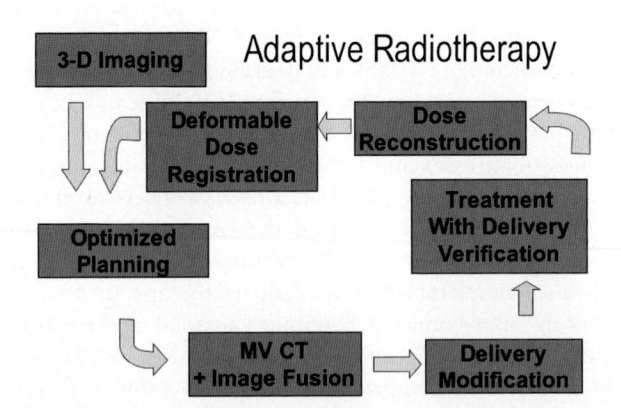

Fig. 2. Flow diagram of helical tomotherapy adaptive processes. (*Courtesy of* T.R. Mackie, PhD, Madison, WI.)

is the inability to correct for organ displacement or distortion that occurs during treatment and over the course of the prescribed protocol. Regardless of how wonderful a dose-volume histogram (graphic representation of dose delivered to outlined volumes of organs at risk and tumor) may look, the clinical application of the treatment plan must be applied with care [42]. Patient immobilization techniques, such as vacuum-formable mattresses, head frames, and various patient markers, are used to exert as much control over interfraction movements as possible [46,47]. Respiratory monitoring devices may allow for respiratory gating or delivery of radiation therapy during the appropriate phase of respiration as determined from the original treatment plan [42]. Ultimately, the goal of adaptive radiotherapy is to continue improving dose delivery and dose verification such that modifications can be made during the course of therapy, which should optimize targeted radiation therapy.

HELICAL TOMOTHERAPY AND CONFORMAL AVOIDANCE

With the conformal avoidance approach and the organ localization and verification offered by helical tomotherapy, it may be possible to spare critical structures further, particularly those organs located immediately adjacent to the target volume. Returning to the popular theme of head and neck cancer in human radiation oncology, the clinical implementation of helical tomotherapy is occurring in a stepwise fashion. Dosimetric comparisons indicate that helical tomotherapy provides superior dose distributions for head and neck cancers and improved sparing of normal parotid gland tissue as well as ocular structures [48,49]. Early studies evaluating canine patients that had spontaneous nasopharyngeal tumors showed that helical tomotherapy delivered effective therapy without excessive ocular toxicity despite the close proximity of the eyes to the nasal cavities and frontal sinuses (Fig. 3) [50]. Further investigations and follow-up are required for realization of improvements in radiation therapy outcome through the use of helical tomotherapy.

BIOLOGIC ADVANTAGES TO HELICAL TOMOTHERAPY

Adaptive radiation therapy and conformal avoidance represent the physical benefits offered by helical tomotherapy. Once these steps are evaluated and verified, adjustments in dose are likely reasonable subsequent steps to take to improve local control and increase survival, particularly in those tumors that are slow to metastasize but exhibit aggressive and early local recurrence. Dose escalation with the preservation of normal tissue integrity is postulated to improve control; however, this has not always yielded improved survival, likely for numerous reasons, including increased late tissue toxicity and prolongation of treatment duration [42]. Prolonged fractionation schedules that deliver an increased total dose to tumor likely increase tumor cell death, but accelerated repopulation likely limits this increase in clonogenic death [42]. For tumors with short potential doubling times, it is likely better to accelerate the treatment protocol or increase the dose per fraction. The limiting factors with accelerated and hypofractionated radiation therapy protocols

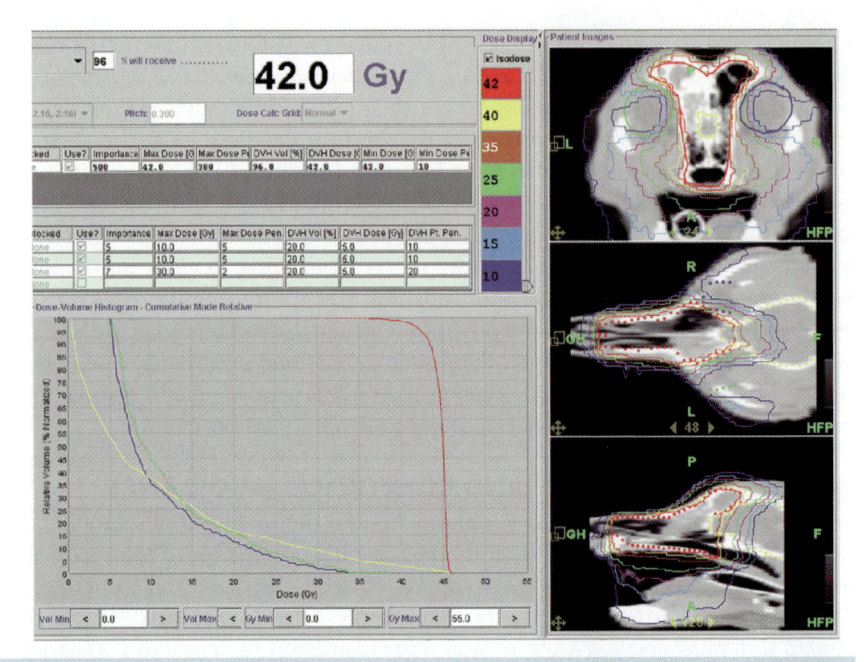

Fig. 3. Helical tomotherapy IMRT treatment plan with dose-volume histogram for a dog with a nasal tumor. Isodose distributions and dose-volume histogram are shown, which are typical for the treatment of the 31 dogs with nasal tumors using helical tomotherapy. The IMRT plan was designed and delivered using the helical tomotherapy treatment planning software and machine. On the right from top to bottom are the axial CT image, the reconstructed dorsal plane CT image, and the reconstructed sagittal CT image. The red line represents the PTV, and the green, blue, and yellow lines represent the right eye, left eye, and brain, respectively. Note the homogeneous dose to the PTV and the sparing of the adjacent eyes and rostral brain.

include increased acute toxicity and greater likelihood of late toxicity, respectively. With the advent of image-guided and adaptive helical tomotherapy, normal tissue toxicity can be limited and increasingly larger doses may be given per fraction, thus improving the therapeutic ratio by increasing tumor control probability while maintaining or reducing the risk of late-term radiation effects. At the University of Wisconsin-Madison Comprehensive Cancer Center, researchers have compared helical tomotherapy planning for patients who had non–small-cell lung cancer (NSCLC) with patients treated with conventional 3D techniques. In this evaluation, helical tomotherapy planning demonstrated improved dose distributions with highly conformal isodose lines and sharp dose gradients surrounding the tumor volume [42]. Compared with conventional 3D treatment plans, tomotherapy plans yield more homogeneous coverage of the tumor volume and lower doses delivered to the surrounding normal lung, esophagus, and spinal cord [42]. When combined with the MVCT verification processes to prevent geographic miss and improve target localization, helical tomotherapy planning should allow significant dose escalation beyond what was possible with 3D conformal radiation therapy and even with conventional IMRT plans.

Highly conformal radiation therapy and the opportunity for dose escalation have major implications for veterinary patients, similar to human patients. Neoplasms, such as intra-abdominal sarcomas, retroperitoneal sarcomas, primary pulmonary carcinomas, pancreatic or gastric carcinomas, nasal and paranasal tumors, and cerebrospinal tumors, may be more effectively controlled by dose escalations while preserving surrounding critical tissues. In such cases as primary lung tumors with tracheobronchial lymph node involvement, both sites could be irradiated after surgery or before surgery in an attempt to gain improved control, which might translate to improved survival. Tomotherapy also lends itself to synchronous boost strategies, because multiple targets can be treated during rotational delivery. This may afford further advantages in shortening treatment duration, reducing the number of general anesthetic episodes, and reducing treatment cost for veterinary patients. Interestingly, a major driver for radiation therapy cost in the United States is the duration of treatment, and a schedule increase from 6 weeks to 10 weeks, as would be expected with conventional dose escalation, increases the cost of therapy by 40% to 50% [51,52]. The use of helical tomotherapy in human radiation oncology may reduce the number of treatments by allowing accelerated protocols [42]. The cost of treatment is lower for veterinary patients, in part because of the compromise between increased dose per fraction compared with human radiation protocols and the need for daily general anesthesia. Unfortunately, lower costs are unlikely to be incurred by veterinary clients with the development of helical tomotherapy unless some form of external support is provided. The helical tomotherapy unit, software, support, and service contract increase the cost of therapy. Nevertheless, because it seems to offer superior therapy, and as awareness of adaptive radiation therapy grows, clients are likely to seek improved therapy for their pets in the future.

POTENTIAL NEGATIVE IMPLICATIONS OF HELICAL TOMOTHERAPY AND INTENSITY-MODULATED RADIATION THERAPY

Although the potential benefits of helical tomotherapy are numerous, there are likely some negative implications of this technique that may be realized as more research and data are gathered over the coming decade. With the transition from 3D conformal radiation therapy to IMRT, an increasing number of treatment fields are involved, such that a larger volume of normal tissue is exposed to lower radiation doses. Reducing the dose theoretically limits the risk of late-term complications for all situations except one: secondary cancer induction. It is predicted that IMRT is likely to almost double the incidence of second malignancies (carcinomas) compared with conventional radiation therapy from approximately 1% to 1.75% for patients surviving 10 years after therapy [53]. This estimate of increased incidence pertains to 6-MV linear accelerators, and the authors of this article acknowledge that the estimates for second cancer formation are much higher for 18-MV linear accelerators and tomotherapy [53]. The increased risk of second cancer formation is acceptable in older patients because it is likely balanced by increased local tumor control and decreased toxicity [54]. The impact on pediatric patients may be more marked, however; children are more sensitive to radiation-induced cancers, genetic susceptibility may play an important role in further increasing the likelihood of secondary malignancy, and radiation scatter is more important in a child's body compared with that of a larger adult [54]. This impact may translate into similar risks for canine and feline patients, particularly if we are able to control localized tumors better and prolong survival. The overall lifespan of our companion animal patients is shorter than that of human patients, however. Currently, veterinary oncologists tend to report a rate of significant (clinically relevant) late toxicity of less than 5%, but this may change if we improve local tumor control and overall survival. As IMRT and helical tomotherapy are increasingly used clinically, accrued data should illustrate the true risks and benefits of therapy.

Another complication of therapy is the likelihood of technical difficulties, particularly as the tomotherapy unit is initially being used for treatment. There is a steep learning curve for the operator, and patience is certainly a virtue in the initial phases of implementation. Technical and medical physics support is crucial.

SUMMARY

IMRT, especially image-guided IMRT as represented by helical tomotherapy, is a novel approach to therapy and is rapidly evolving. Tomotherapy offers MVCT image guidance and setup verification as well as an infinite number of beam origins to allow for targeted and precise delivery of radiation therapy. Adaptive radiation therapy and conformal avoidance are possible with helical tomotherapy, which offers opportunities for improved local tumor control, decreased normal tissue toxicity, and improved survival and quality of life. Human and veterinary patients should benefit from the continued development of this radiation delivery technique, and data over the next several years should be crucial in determining its true benefit. Tomotherapy most certainly is a stepping stone to further physical and biologic advancements in the treatment of cancer and could potentially alter the current paradigm in radiation oncology.

Acknowledgments

The authors thank Drs. Minesh Mehta, Hazim Jaradat, and Thomas R. Mackie for their persistent assistance and support.

References

[1] Hall EJ, Giaccia AJ. Clinical response of normal tissues. In: Hall EJ, Giaccia AJ, editors. Radiobiology for the radiologist. 6th edition. Philadelphia: Lippincott Williams & Wilkins; 2006. p. 327–48.

[2] Hall EJ, Giaccia AJ. Time, dose, and fractionation in radiotherapy. In: Hall EJ, Giaccia AJ, editors. Radiobiology for the radiologist. 6th edition. Philadelphia: Lippincott Williams & Wilkins; 2006. p. 378–97.

[3] Hill RP, Bristow RG. The scientific basis of radiotherapy. In: Tannock IF, Hill RP, Bristow RG, et al, editors. The basic science of oncology. 4th edition. New York: McGraw-Hill; 2005. p. 289–321.

[4] Takahashi S. Conformation radiotherapy—rotation techniques as applied to radiography and radiotherapy of cancer. Acta Radiol 1965;242(Suppl):1–142.

[5] Mackie TR, Kapatoes J, Ruchala K, et al. Image guidance for precise conformal radiotherapy. Int J Radiat Oncol Biol Phys 2003;56:89–105.

[6] Prado KL, Prado C. Dose distributions. In: Washington CM, Leaver D, editors. Principles and practice of radiation therapy. 2nd edition. St Louis (MO): Mosby; 2004. p. 505–27.

[7] Lee CB, Stinchcombe TE, Rosenman JG, et al. Therapeutic advances in local-regional therapy for stage III non-small-cell lung cancer: evolving role of dose-escalated conformal (3-dimensional) radiation therapy. Clin Lung Cancer 2006;8:195–202.

[8] Ceha HM, van Tienhoven G, Gouma DJ, et al. Feasibility and efficacy of high dose conformal radiotherapy for patients with locally advanced pancreatic carcinoma. Cancer 2000;89:2222–9.

[9] Hanks GE, Hanlon AL, Schultheiss TE, et al. Dose escalation with 3D conformal treatment: five year outcomes, treatment optimization, and future directions. Int J Radiat Oncol Biol Phys 1998;41:501–10.

[10] Purdy JA. Current ICRU definitions of volumes: limitations and future directions. Semin Radiat Oncol 2004;14:27–40.

[11] Nutting CM, Convery DJ, Cosgrove VP, et al. Reduction of small and large bowel irradiation using an optimized intensity-modulated pelvic radiotherapy technique in patients with prostate cancer. Int J Radiat Oncol Biol Phys 2000;48:649–56.

[12] Pirzkall A, Carol M, Lohr F, et al. Comparison of intensity-modulated radiotherapy with conventional conformal radiotherapy for complex-shaped tumors. Int J Radiat Oncol Biol Phys 2000;48:1371–80.

[13] IMRT Collaborative Working Group. Intensity-modulated radiotherapy. Current status and issues of interest. Int J Radiat Oncol Biol Phys 2001;51:880–914.

[14] Verhey LJ. Comparison of three-dimensional conformal radiation therapy and intensity-modulated radiation therapy systems. Semin Radiat Oncol 1999;9:78–98.

[15] Cheng JC, Wu JK, Huang CM, et al. Dosimetric analysis and comparison of three-dimensional conformal radiotherapy and intensity-modulated radiation therapy for patients with hepatocellular carcinoma and radiation-induced liver disease. Int J Radiat Oncol Biol Phys 2003;56:229–334.

[16] Kam MK, Chau RM, Suen J, et al. Intensity-modulated radiotherapy in nasopharyngeal carcinoma: dosimetric advantage over conventional plans and feasibility of dose escalation. Int J Radiat Oncol Biol Phys 2003;56:145–57.

[17] Schwarz M, Alber M, Lebesque JV, et al. Dose heterogeneity in the target volume and intensity-modulated radiotherapy to escalate the dose in the treatment of non-small-cell lung cancer. Int J Radiat Oncol Biol Phys 2005;62:561–70.

[18] Grills IS, Yan D, Martinez AA, et al. Potential for reduced toxicity and dose escalation in the treatment of inoperable non-small-cell lung cancer: a comparison of intensity-modulated radiation therapy (IMRT), 3D conformal radiation, and elective nodal irradiation. Int J Radiat Oncol Biol Phys 2003;57:875–90.

[19] Mackie TR, Balog J, Ruchala K, et al. Tomotherapy. Semin Radiat Oncol 1999;9:108–17.

[20] Beavis AW. Is tomotherapy the future of IMRT? Br J Radiol 2004;77:285–95.

[21] Chao KS. Protection of salivary function by intensity-modulated radiation therapy in patients with head and neck cancer. Semin Radiat Oncol 2002;12(S1):20–5.

[22] Warde P, O'Sullivan B, Aslanidis J, et al. A phase-III placebo-controlled trial of oral pilocarpine in patients undergoing radiotherapy for head-and-neck cancer. Int J Radiat Oncol Biol Phys 2002;54:9–13.

[23] Scarantino C, LeVeque F, Swann RS, et al. Effect of pilocarpine during radiation therapy: results of RTOG 97-09, a phase III randomized study in head and neck cancer patients. J Support Oncol 2006;4:252–8.

[24] Guchelaar HJ, Vermes A, Meerwaldt JH. Radiation-induced xerostomia: pathophysiology, clinical course and supportive treatment. Support Care Cancer 1997;5:281–8.

[25] Brizol DM, Wasserman TH, Henke M, et al. Phase III randomized trial of amifostine as a radioprotector in head and neck cancer. J Clin Oncol 2000;18:3339–45.

[26] Wasserman TH, Brizol DM, Henke K, et al. Influence of intravenous amifostine on xerostomia, tumor control, and survival after radiotherapy for head-and-neck cancer: 2-year follow-up of a prospective, randomized, phase III trial. Int J Radiat Oncol Biol Phys 2005;63:985–90.

[27] Chao KS, Deasy JO, Markman J, et al. A prospective study of salivary function sparing in patients with head-and-neck cancers receiving intensity-modulated or three-dimensional radiation therapy: initial results. Int J Radiat Oncol Biol Phys 2001;49:907–16.

[28] Chao KS, Ozyigit G, Blanco A, et al. Intensity-modulated radiation therapy for oropharyngeal carcinoma: impact of tumor volume. Int J Radiat Oncol Biol Phys 2004;59:43–50.

[29] Parliament MB, Scrimger RA, Anderson SG, et al. Preservation of oral health-related quality of life and salivary flow rates after inverse-planned intensity- modulated radiotherapy (IMRT) for head-and-neck cancer. Int J Radiat Oncol Biol Phys 2004;58:663–73.

[30] Munter MW, Karger CP, Hoffner SG, et al. Evaluation of salivary gland function after treatment of head-and-neck tumors with intensity-modulated radiotherapy by quantitative pertechnetate scintigraphy. Int J Radiat Oncol Biol Phys 2004;58:175–84.

[31] Jabbari S, Kim HM, Feng M, et al. Matched case-control study of quality of life and xerostomia after intensity-modulated radiotherapy or standard radiotherapy for head-and-neck cancer: initial report. Int J Radiat Oncol Biol Phys 2005;63:725–31.

[32] MacEwen EG, Withrow SJ, Patnaik AK. Nasal tumors in the dog: retrospective evaluation of diagnosis, prognosis, and treatment. J Am Vet Med Assoc 1977;170:45–8.

[33] Beck ER, Withrow SJ. Tumors of the canine nasal cavity. Vet Clin North Am Small Anim Pract 1985;15:521–33.

[34] Adams WM, Withrow SJ, Walshaw R, et al. Radiotherapy of malignant nasal tumors in 67 dogs. J Am Vet Med Assoc 1987;191:311–5.

[35] Thrall DE, Harvey CE. Radiotherapy of malignant nasal tumors in 21 dogs. J Am Vet Med Assoc 1983;183:663–6.

[36] Theon AP, Madewell BR, Harb MF, et al. Megavoltage irradiation of neoplasms of the nasal and paranasal cavities in 77 dogs. J Am Vet Med Assoc 1993;202:1469–75.

[37] Adams WM, Miller PE, Vail DM, et al. An accelerated technique for irradiation of malignant canine nasal and paranasal sinus tumors. Vet Radiol Ultrasound 1998;39:475–81.

[38] Adams WM, Bjorling DE, McAnulty JF, et al. Outcome of accelerated radiotherapy alone or accelerated radiotherapy followed by exenteration of the nasal cavity in dogs with intranasal neoplasia: 53 cases (1990–2002). J Am Vet Med Assoc 2005;227:936–41.

[39] Roberts SM, Lavach JD, Severin GA, et al. Ophthalmic complications following megavoltage irradiation of the nasal and paranasal cavities in the dogs. J Am Vet Med Assoc 1987;100:43–7.

[40] Forrest LJ, Mackie TR, Ruchala K, et al. The utility of megavoltage computed tomography images from a helical tomotherapy system for setup verification purposes. Int J Radiat Oncol Biol Phys 2004;60:1639–44.

[41] Mackie TR, Holmes TW, Swerdloff S, et al. Tomotherapy: a new concept for the delivery of conformal radiotherapy. Med Phys 1993;20:1709–19.

[42] Welsh JS, Lock M, Harari PM, et al. Clinical implementation of adaptive helical tomotherapy: a unique approach to image-guided intensity modulated radiotherapy. Technol Cancer Res Treat 2006;5:465–80.
[43] Welsh JS, Bradley K, Manon R, et al. Megavoltage CT imaging for adaptive helical tomotherapy of lung cancer. Clin Lung Cancer 2004;5:303–6.
[44] Yan D, Lockman D, Brabbins D, et al. An off-line strategy for constructing a patient-specific planning target volume in adaptive treatment process for prostate cancer. Int J Radiat Oncol Biol Phys 2000;48:289–302.
[45] Kapatoes JM, Olivera G, Balog JP, et al. On the accuracy and effectiveness of dose reconstruction for tomotherapy. Phys Med Biol 2001;46:943–66.
[46] Green EM, Forrest LJ, Adams WM. A vacuum-formable mattress for veterinary radiotherapy positioning: comparison with conventional methods. Vet Radiol Ultrasound 2003;44: 476–9.
[47] Bley CR, Blattman H, Roos M, et al. Assessment of a radiotherapy patient immobilization device using single plane port radiographs and a remote computed tomography scanner. Vet Radiol Ultrasound 2003;44:470–5.
[48] van Vulpen M, Field C, Raaijmakers CP, et al. Comparing step-and-shoot IMRT with dynamic helical tomotherapy IMRT plans for head-and-neck cancer. Int J Radiat Oncol Biol Phys 2005;62:1535–9.
[49] Sheng K, Molloy JA, Larner JM, et al. A dosimetric comparison of non-coplanar IMRT versus helical tomotherapy for nasal cavity and paranasal sinus cancer. Radiother Oncol 2007; 82:174–8.
[50] Forrest LJ, Lawrence JA, Miller PE, et al. Ocular sparing using image-guided helical tomotherapy (IGHT) in spontaneous sino-nasal tumors in dogs. Int J Radiat Oncol Biol Phys 2006;66:S425.
[51] Horwitz EM, Hanlon AL, Pinover WH, et al. The cost-effectiveness of 3D conformal radiation therapy compared with conventional techniques for patients with clinically localized prostate cancer. Int J Radiat Oncol Biol Phys 1999;45:1219–26.
[52] Legorreta AP, Brooks RH, Leibowitz AN, et al. Cost of breast cancer treatment. A 4-year longitudinal study. Arch Intern Med 1996;156:2197–201.
[53] Hall EJ, Wuu CS. Radiation induced second cancers: the impact of 3DCRT and IMRT. Int J Radiat Oncol Biol Phys 2003;56:83–8.
[54] Hall EJ. The inaugural Frank Ellis Lecture—iatrogenic cancer: the impact of intensity-modulated radiotherapy. Clin Oncol (R Coll Radiol) 2006;18:277–82.

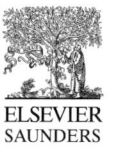

VETERINARY CLINICS
SMALL ANIMAL PRACTICE

INDEX

A

AB1010, 1127

Abdominal neoplasia, MRI of, 1066

Active controls, defined, 1053

Acute systemic inflammatory reaction, bisphosphonates and, 1097

Adaptive radiotherapy, 1158–1159

Adaptive trial designs, defined, 1053

AKC-CHF. See *American Kennel Club–Canine Health Foundation (AKC-CHF)*.

American College of Veterinary Internal Medicine, 1028

American College of Veterinary Radiology, 1028

American Kennel Club–Canine Health Foundation (AKC-CHF), 1026

Aminobisphosphonate(s), in cancer-bearing dogs and cats, 1102–1105

Animal Medical Center, DNA vaccine program for melanoma at, 1115

Antiangiogenesis, bisphosphonates and, 1099–1100

Antibody(ies)
 immunotoxin-conjugated, 1144
 monoclonal, unconjugated, 1143–1144
 radionuclide-conjugated, 1144–1145

Anticancer vaccines, **1111–1119**
 goal for, 1113
 types of, 1113–1115

Antigen(s), cancer testes, 1113–1115

Autophosphorylation, 1121

Avoidance, conformal. See *Conformal avoidance*.

B

Bacillus of Calmette and Guérin and mycobacterial cell wall–DNA complex, 1138–1139

Bayesian adaptive designs, for clinical trials, 1047–1048

Bayesian approach to statistical analysis, defined, 1053

Biologic response modifiers, 1138–1141
 Bacillus of Calmette and Guérin and mycobacterial cell wall–DNA complex, 1138–1139
 liposome-DNA complexes, 1139–1140
 liposome-encapsulated muramyl tripeptide, 1139
 oncolytic viruses, 1140–1141

Bisphosphonate(s)
 absorption of, 1093–1094
 adverse effects of, 1096–1098
 antiresorptive potency of, 1092–1093
 chemical structure of, 1092–1093
 described, 1091–1092
 distribution of, 1094–1095
 excretion of, 1095
 in cancer management, **1091–1110**
  antiangiogenesis, 1099–1100
  anti-invasive effects, 1099
  antiproliferative effects, 1099
  molecular targets, 1098–1100
  therapeutic response assessment, 1100–1102
   bone-specific biochemical methodologies, 1101–1102
   newer radiologic methods, 1100–1101
   traditional radiologic methods, 1100
 mechanism of action of, 1095–1096
 metabolism of, 1095
 pharmacokinetics of, 1093–1095
 terminal elimination of, 1095

Bone pain, osteolytic, aminobisphosphonates in, 1102–1104

B-RAF, 1126

Brain tumors
 CT of, 1061–1063
 MRI of, 1065–1066

Note: Page numbers of article titles are in **boldface** type.

C

Cancer
  clinical trials for
    basic structure of, 1033, 1034
    development and implementation of, **1033–1057**. See also *Clinical trials*.
  head and neck, conformal avoidance and, 1154–1155
  immunotherapy for, **1137–1149**. See also *Immunotherapy*.
  in dogs, problems associated with, 1023–1024
  management of, bisphosphonates in, **1091–1110**. See also *Bisphosphonate(s)*.
  vaccines against, 1113–1117. See also *Anticancer vaccines*.
Cancer immunosurveillance, 1112
Cancer patients, advanced imaging for, **1059–1077**. See also specific modality, e.g., *Computed tomography (CT)*.
  cross-sectional imaging modalities, 1060–1067
  CT, 1060–1064
  MRI, 1065–1067
  PET, 1067–1073
  PET/CT, 1067–1073
  PET/CT fusion, 1069–1070
Cancer testes antigens, 1113–1115
Canine Genome Project, 1025
Cat(s), cancer in, aminobisphosphonates in, 1102–1105
CCOGC. See *Comparative Oncology and Genomics Consortium (CCOGC)*.
Chemotherapy, **1079–1090**
  clinical trials, 1085–1087
  combination therapy, 1085
  dosing, 1080
  metronomic, 1079
    as antiangiogenic strategy, 1082–1085
      circulating endothelial progenitor cells, 1083–1084
      described, 1082–1083
      growth/survival factor modulation, 1084–1085
      selective endothelial cell cytotoxicity, 1083
    pharmacology of, 1081–1082
Circulating endothelial progenitor cells, in metronomic chemotherapy, 1083–1084
Clinical trials
  adaptive designs, 1047
  basic structure of, 1033, 1034
  Bayesian adaptive designs, 1047–1048
  cancer-related, development and implementation of, **1033–1057**
  chemotherapy-related, 1085–1087
  crossover trials, 1051–1052
  enrichment, 1050–1051
  informed consent for, 1052
  noninferiority trials, 1051
  phase 0, defined, 1054
  phase combinations, 1049–1050
  phase I, 1035–1038
    candidates for, 1036
    defined, 1054
    described, 1035–1036
    dose escalation strategies, 1036–1038
    starting dose in, setting of, 1036
  phase II, 1038–1043
    controlled, 1041–1043
    defined, 1054
    described, 1038–1040
    end points of activity/efficacy, 1040–1041
  phase III, 1043–1044
    defined, 1054
  phase IV, 1044
    defined, 1054
  phase 0, 1045–1046
  randomization in, 1044–1045
  randomized discontinuation trials, 1048–1049
  standard designs for, modifications/alternatives to, 1044–1052
  stopping rules in, 1047
  terminology related to, 1053–1055
  traditional drug development flow in, 1035–1044
Cohort study, defined, 1053
Communication
  with oncology clients, **1013–1022**
    breaking news/presenting diagnosis, 1015–1016
    end-of-life decisions, 1019–1020
    euthanasia, 1020–1021
    offering options, 1016–1018
    providing support, 1018–1019
    responding to client emotion, 1016
Communication skills, review of, 1013–1015
Comparative oncology, **1023–1032**
  cancer in dogs and, 1024–1029
Comparative Oncology and Genomics Consortium (CCOGC), 1028
Comparative Oncology Program (COP), 1028
Comparative Oncology Trials Consortium (COTC), 1028

INDEX

Computed tomography (CT), for cancer patients, 1060–1064
   clinical applications, 1061–1064
      brain tumors, 1061–1063
      extremity-related neoplasia, 1064
      integumental neoplasia, 1064
      intra-abdominal neoplasia, 1064
      intrathoracic neoplasia, 1063–1064
      mediastinal tumors, 1064
      metastatic lung disease, 1064
      nasal tumors, 1063
      non–CNS head and neck tumors, 1063
      oral cavity tumors, 1063
      primary lung tumors, 1063–1064
      skull tumors, 1063
      spinal/paraspinal tumors, 1061–1063
   technical advances in, 1060–1061
Conditional power, defined, 1053
Conformal avoidance
   described, 1153–1154
   helical tomotherapy and, 1159
   human head and neck cancer and, 1154–1155
   IMRT and, 1152–1153
Control(s), active, defined, 1053
COP. See *Comparative Oncology Program (COP)*.
COTC. See *Comparative Oncology Trials Consortium (COTC)*.
Crossover trials, 1051–1052
Cross-sectional imaging modalities, for cancer patients, 1060–1067
CT. See *Computed tomography (CT)*.
Cytokine therapy, 1141–1143
   IL-2, 1141–1142
   IL-12, 1142
   tumor necrosis factor-α, 1142–1143
Cytoplasmic kinases, 1122

D

DNA vaccine program, for melanoma, at Animal Medical Center, 1115
Dog(s), cancer in
   aminobisphonates in, 1102–1105
   comparative oncology and, 1024–1029
   problems associated with, 1023–1024

E

EGFR, 1127
Electrolyte(s), abnormalities of, bisphosphonates and, 1098
End-of-life decisions, communicating with oncology clients about, 1019–1020
Enrichment, defined, 1053
Enrichment clinical trials, 1050–1051
Euthanasia, communicating with oncology client about, 1020–1021
Extremity(ies), neoplasia of
   CT of, 1064
   MRI of, 1066–1067
Eye(s), bisphosphonates effects on, 1097

F

First-in-species trial, defined, 1053
Frequentist approach to statistical analysis, defined, 1053
Futility analysis, defined, 1053

G

Gastrointestinal tract, bisphosphonates effects on, 1096
Gefitinib, 1125–1126
Gleevec, 1123–1125, 1127–1128
Growth/survival factor modulation, in metronomic chemotherapy, 1084–1085

H

Head and neck cancer, human, conformal avoidance and, 1154–1155
Head and neck tumors, non–CNS
   CT of, 1063
   MRI of, 1066
Heat shock protein 90 (HSP90) inhibitors, 1128–1129
Helical tomotherapy, **1151–1165**
   biologic advantages to, 1159–1161
   conformal avoidance and, 1159
   image-guided radiation therapy and, 1155–1157
   negative implications of, 1161–1162
Histone deacetylase inhibitors, 1131–1132
HSP90 inhibitors. See *Heat shock protein 90 (HSP90) inhibitors*.
Hypercalcemia, tumor-induced, management of, aminobisphonates in, 1104–1105
Hypothesis(es), null, defined, 1054

I

IL. See *Interleukin(s)*.
Image-guided radiation therapy, helical tomotherapy and, 1155–1157
Imaging, advanced, for cancer patients, **1059–1077**. See also specific modality and *Cancer patients, advanced imaging for*.

Immune responses, described, 1112
Immunity, defined, 1111
Immunology, tumor-related, 1111–1113
Immunosurveillance, cancer, 1112
Immunotherapy, **1137–1149**
    future challenges for, 1145–1146
    nonspecific tumor, 1113, 1137–1143
        biologic response modifiers, 1138–1141
            Bacillus of Calmette and Guérin and mycobacterial cell wall–DNA complex, 1138–1139
            liposome-DNA complexes, 1139–1140
            liposome-encapsulated muramyl tripeptide, 1139
            oncolytic viruses, 1140–1141
        cytokine therapy, 1141–1143
            IL-2, 1141–1142
            IL-12, 1142
            tumor necrosis factor-α, 1142–1143
    tumor-specific, 1143–1145
        immunotoxin-conjugated antibodies, 1144
        radionuclide-conjugated antibodies, 1144–1145
        unconjugated monoclonal antibodies, 1143–1144
Immunotoxin-conjugated antibodies, 1144
IMRT. See *Intensity-modulated radiation therapy (IMRT)*.
Integument, neoplasia of
    CT of, 1064
    MRI of, 1066–1067
Intensity-modulated radiation therapy (IMRT), **1151–1165**
    conformal avoidance and, 1152–1153
    negative implications of, 1161–1162
Intention-to-treat analysis, defined, 1054
Interleukin(s)
    IL-2, 1141–1142
    IL-12, 1142
Interviewing techniques, examples of, 1014
Intra-abdominal neoplasia, CT of, 1064
Intrathoracic neoplasia, CT of, 1063–1064

K

Kinase(s)
    cytoplasmic, 1122
    protein, 1121–1122
        dysfunction of, 1123
    tyrosine, 1122
Kinase inhibitors, 1126–1128
    human experience with, 1121–1126
Kit, 1126–1127

L

Liposome-DNA complexes, 1139–1140
Liposome-encapsulated muramyl tripeptide, 1139
Lung disease, metastatic, CT of, 1064
Lung tumors, primary, CT of, 1063–1064

M

MAF. See *Morris Animal Foundation (MAF)*.
Magnetic resonance imaging (MRI), for cancer patients, 1065–1067
    clinical applications
        abdominal neoplasia, 1066
        brain tumors, 1065–1066
        extremity-related neoplasia, 1066–1067
        non–CNS head and neck tumors, 1066
    clinical applications of, 1065–1067
    MRI of, integumental neoplasia, 1066–1067
    technical advances in, 1065
Mandible, osteonecrosis of, bisphosphonates and, 1098
Maxilla, osteonecrosis of, bisphosphonates and, 1098
Maximum tolerated dose (MTD), 1080
Mediastinal tumors, CT of, 1064
Melanoma, DNA vaccine program for, at Animal Medical Center, 1115
Memorial Sloan-Kettering Cancer Center, 1115
Met, 1127
Metastatic lung disease, CT of, 1064
Monoclonal antibodies, unconjugated, 1143–1144
Morris Animal Foundation (MAF), 1026
MRI. See *Magnetic resonance imaging (MRI)*.
MTD. See *Maximum tolerated dose (MTD)*.

N

Nasal tumors, CT of, 1063
National Cancer Institute, 1028
Neck cancer, human, conformal avoidance and, 1154–1155

INDEX

Neck tumors, non–CNS
  CT of, 1063
  MRI of, 1066
Nephrotic syndrome, bisphosphonates and, 1097–1098
Noninferiority trials, 1051
Nonspecific tumor immunotherapy, 1137–1143. See also *Immunotherapy, nonspecific tumor.*
Null hypothesis, defined, 1054

O

Oncolytic viruses, 1140–1141
Oral cavity, tumors of, CT of, 1063
Osteolytic bone pain, aminobisphosphonates in, 1102–1104
Osteonecrosis, of maxilla and mandible, bisphosphonates and, 1098

P

Paraspinal tumors
  CT of, 1061–1063
  MRI of, 1065–1066
PET. See *Positron emission tomography (PET).*
PET/CT. See *Positron emission tomography (PET)/CT.*
Phase 0 trials, 1045–1046
  defined, 1054
Phase I trials, 1035–1038
  defined, 1054
Phase II trials, 1038–1043
  defined, 1054
Phase III trials, 1043–1044
  defined, 1054
Phase IV trials, 1044
  defined, 1054
Phosphatidyl inositol 3 kinase (PI3K), 1122
PI3K. See *Phosphatidyl inositol 3 kinase (PI3K).*
Positron emission tomography (PET)
  for cancer patients, 1067–1073
    clinical applications, 1071–1073
    image interpretation, 1070–1071
    practical aspects, 1070
    technical aspects, 1067–1071
  physics of, 1067–1069
Positron emission tomography (PET)/CT, for cancer patients, 1067–1073
  clinical applications, 1071–1073
  image interpretation, 1070–1071
  practical aspects, 1070
  technical aspects, 1067–1071
Positron emission tomography (PET)/CT fusion, for cancer patients, 1069–1070

Positron-emitting radiopharmaceutic agents, physics of, 1067–1069
Power, conditional, defined, 1053
Predictive factors, defined, 1054
Prognostic factors, defined, 1054
Prospective clinical trials, defined, 1054
Proteasome inhibitors, 1129–1131
Protein kinases, 1121–1122
  dysfunction of, 1123

R

Radiation therapy
  adaptive, 1158–1159
  image-guided, helical tomotherapy and, 1155–1157
  intensity-modulated, **1151–1165**. See also *Intensity-modulated radiation therapy (IMRT).*
  three-dimensional conformal, 1151–1152
Radionuclide-conjugated antibodies, 1144–1145
Randomization
  defined, 1054
  in clinical trials, 1044–1045
  unbalanced, defined, 1055
Randomized discontinuation trials, 1048–1049
RAS-RAF-MEK-ERK/p38/JNK families, 1122
Receptor tyrosine kinases (RTKs), 1122
Renal failure, acute and chronic, bisphosphonates and, 1097
Retrospective studies, defined, 1054
RTKs. See *Receptor tyrosine kinases (RTKs).*

S

Selective endothelial cell cytotoxicity, in metronomic chemotherapy, 1083
Skull tumors, CT of, 1063
Small molecule inhibitors
  AB1010, 1127
  EGFR, 1127
  gefitinib, 1125–1126
  Gleevec, 1123–1125, 1127–1128
  histone deacetylase inhibitors, 1131–1132
  HSP90 inhibitors, 1128–1129
  kinase inhibitors, human experience with, 1121–1126
  Kit, 1126–1127
  Met, 1127
  proteasome inhibitors, 1129–1131
  role of, **1121–1136**

Small (continued)
    SU11654, 1127
    SUTENT, 1125
Spinal/paraspinal tumors
    CT of, 1061–1063
    MRI of, 1065–1066
Standard of care, defined, 1054
Statistical analysis
    Bayesian approach to, defined, 1053
    frequentist approach to, defined, 1053
Stochastic curtailing, defined, 1054
Stopping rules
    defined, 1054
    in clinical trials, 1047
Stratification, defined, 1054
SU11654, 1127
SUTENT, 1125

T

Three-dimensional conformal radiation therapy, 1151–1152
Tomotherapy, helical, **1151–1165**. See also *Helical tomotherapy*.
Tumor(s)
    brain
        CT of, 1061–1063
        MRI of, 1065–1066
    head and neck, non–CNS
        CT of, 1063
        MRI of, 1066
    hypercalcemia due to, management of, aminobisphosphonates in, 1104–1105
    immunology of, 1111–1113
    immunotherapy for, nonspecific, 1113
    lung, primary, CT of, 1063–1064
    mediastinal, CT of, 1064
    nasal, CT of, 1063
    oral cavity, CT of, 1063
    skull, CT of, 1063
    spinal/paraspinal
        CT of, 1061–1063
        MRI of, 1065–1066
Tumor necrosis factor-α, 1142–1143
Tumor-specific immunotherapy, 1143–1145. See also *Immunotherapy, tumor-specific*.
Type I error, defined, 1054
Type II error, defined, 1054
Tyrosine kinases, 1122

U

Unbalanced randomization, defined, 1055
Unconjugated monoclonal antibodies, 1143–1144

V

Vaccine(s), anticancer, **1111–1119**. See also *Anticancer vaccines*.
VCOG. See *Veterinary Co-Operative Oncology Group (VCOG)*.
VCOG-CTCAE. See *Veterinary Cooperative Oncology Group Common Terminology Criteria for Adverse Events (VCOG-CTCAE)*.
VCS. See *Veterinary Cancer Society (VCS)*.
Veterinary Cancer Society (VCS), 1028
Veterinary Co-Operative Oncology Group (VCOG), 1028
Veterinary Cooperative Oncology Group Common Terminology Criteria for Adverse Events (VCOG-CTCAE), 1037
Virus(es), oncolytic, 1140–1141

Moving?

Make sure your subscription moves with you!

To notify us of your new address, find your **Clinics Account Number** (located on your mailing label above your name), and contact customer service at:

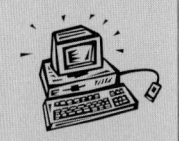

E-mail: elspcs@elsevier.com

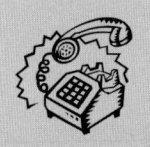

800-654-2452 (subscribers in the U.S. & Canada)
407-345-4000 (subscribers outside of the U.S. & Canada)

Fax number: 407-363-9661

Elsevier Periodicals Customer Service
6277 Sea Harbor Drive
Orlando, FL 32887-4800

*To ensure uninterrupted delivery of your subscription, please notify us at least 4 weeks in advance of move.

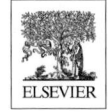

ELSEVIER

United States Postal Service
Statement of Ownership, Management, and Circulation
(All Periodicals Publications Except Requestor Publications)

1. Publication Title	2. Publication Number	3. Filing Date
Veterinary Clinics of North America: Small Animal Practice	0 0 3 - 1 5 0	9/14/07

4. Issue Frequency	5. Number of Issues Published Annually	6. Annual Subscription Price
Jan, Mar, May, Jul, Sep, Nov	6	$187.00

7. Complete Mailing Address of Known Office of Publication (Not printer) (Street, city, county, state, and ZIP+4)

Elsevier Inc.
360 Park Avenue South
New York, NY 10010-1710

Contact Person: Stephen Bushing
Telephone (Include area code): 215-239-3688

8. Complete Mailing Address of Headquarters or General Business Office of Publisher (Not printer)

Elsevier Inc., 360 Park Avenue South, New York, NY 10010-1710

9. Full Names and Complete Mailing Addresses of Publisher, Editor, and Managing Editor (Do not leave blank)

Publisher (Name and complete mailing address)

John Schrefer, Elsevier, Inc., 1600 John F. Kennedy Blvd. Suite 1800, Philadelphia, PA 19103-2899

Editor (Name and complete mailing address)

John Vassallo, Elsevier, Inc., 1600 John F. Kennedy Blvd. Suite 1800, Philadelphia, PA 19103-2899

Managing Editor (Name and complete mailing address)

Catherine Bewick, Elsevier, Inc., 1600 John F. Kennedy Blvd. Suite 1800, Philadelphia, PA 19103-2899

10. Owner (Do not leave blank. If the publication is owned by a corporation, give the name and address of the corporation immediately followed by the names and addresses of all stockholders owning or holding 1 percent or more of the total amount of stock. If not owned by a corporation, give the names and addresses of the individual owners. If owned by a partnership or other unincorporated firm, give its name and address as well as those of each individual owner. If the publication is published by a nonprofit organization, give its name and address.)

Full Name	Complete Mailing Address
Wholly owned subsidiary of	4520 East-West Highway
Reed/Elsevier, US holdings	Bethesda, MD 20814

11. Known Bondholders, Mortgagees, and Other Security Holders Owning or Holding 1 Percent or More of Total Amount of Bonds, Mortgages, or Other Securities. If none, check box — None

Full Name	Complete Mailing Address
N/A	

12. Tax Status (For completion by nonprofit organizations authorized to mail at nonprofit rates) (Check one)
The purpose, function, and nonprofit status of this organization and the exempt status for federal income tax purposes:
☒ Has Not Changed During Preceding 12 Months
☐ Has Changed During Preceding 12 Months (Publisher must submit explanation of change with this statement)

PS Form 3526, September 2006 (Page 1 of 3 (Instructions Page 3)) PSN 7530-01-000-9931 PRIVACY NOTICE: See our Privacy policy in www.usps.com

---

13. Publication Title	14. Issue Date for Circulation Data Below
Veterinary Clinics of North America: Small Animal Practice	September 2007

15. Extent and Nature of Circulation	Average No. Copies Each Issue During Preceding 12 Months	No. Copies of Single Issue Published Nearest to Filing Date
a. Total Number of Copies (Net press run)	3983	3800
b. Paid Circulation (By Mail and Outside the Mail) (1) Mailed Outside-County Paid Subscriptions Stated on PS Form 3541. (Include paid distribution above nominal rate, advertiser's proof copies, and exchange copies)	2360	2321
(2) Mailed In-County Paid Subscriptions Stated on PS Form 3541 (Include paid distribution above nominal rate, advertiser's proof copies, and exchange copies)		
(3) Paid Distribution Outside the Mails Including Sales Through Dealers and Carriers, Street Vendors, Counter Sales, and Other Paid Distribution Outside USPS®	580	599
(4) Paid Distribution by Other Classes Mailed Through the USPS (e.g. First-Class Mail®)		
c. Total Paid Distribution (Sum of 15b (1), (2), (3), and (4))	2940	2920
d. Free or Nominal Rate Distribution (By Mail and Outside the Mail) (1) Free or Nominal Rate Outside-County Copies Included on PS Form 3541	161	150
(2) Free or Nominal Rate In-County Copies Included on PS Form 3541		
(3) Free or Nominal Rate Copies Mailed at Other Classes Mailed Through the USPS (e.g. First-Class Mail)		
(4) Free or Nominal Rate Distribution Outside the Mail (Carriers or other means)		
e. Total Free or Nominal Rate Distribution (Sum of 15d (1), (2), (3) and (4))	161	150
f. Total Distribution (Sum of 15c and 15e)	3101	3070
g. Copies not Distributed (See instructions to publishers #4 (page #3))	882	730
h. Total (Sum of 15f and g)	3983	3800
i. Percent Paid (15c divided by 15f times 100)	94.81%	95.11%

16. Publication of Statement of Ownership
If the publication is a general publication, publication of this statement is required. Will be printed in the November 2007 issue of this publication. ☒ Publication not required

17. Signature and Title of Editor, Publisher, Business Manager, or Owner

[signed] — Executive Director of Subscription Services

Date: September 14, 2007

I certify that all information furnished on this form is true and complete. I understand that anyone who furnishes false or misleading information on this form or who omits material or information requested on the form may be subject to criminal sanctions (including fines and imprisonment) and/or civil sanctions (including civil penalties).

PS Form 3526, September 2006 (Page 2 of 3)

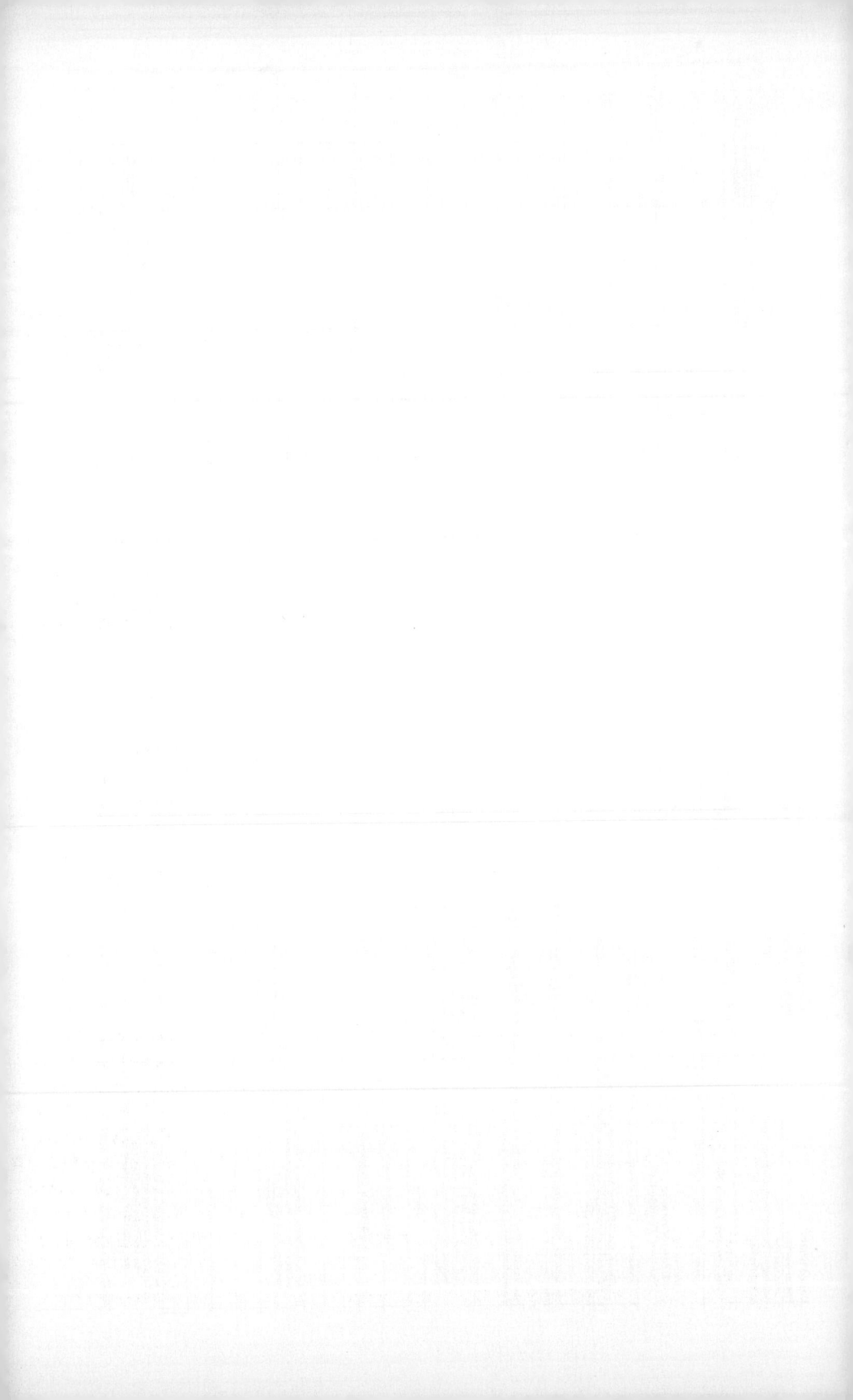